CONQUERING
HEADACHE

SECOND REVISED EDITION

An Illustrated Guide to Understanding
The Treatment and Control of Headache

ALAN RAPOPORT, MD
FRED SHEFTELL, MD

D1466722

1998
Empowering Press, Hamilton, Canada

Second Revised Edition
Copyright © 1998, Alan M. Rapoport and Fred D. Sheftell
All rights reserved.

Canadian Cataloguing in Publication Data

Rapoport, Alan M., 1942 –
    Conquering headache: an illustrated guide to understanding and control of headache

Includes index.
ISBN 1-896998-00-3

1. Headache — Popular works.   I. Sheftell, Fred D., 1941 –   II. Title
RB128.R36 1995   616.8'491   C95-930478-9

For distribution information contact the publisher:

Empowering Press
4 Hughson Street South, P.O. Box 620, L.C.D. 1
Hamilton, Ontario, Canada L8N 3K7
Tel: 905-522-7017; Fax: 905-522-7839; e-mail: info@bcdecker.com

The authors and publisher have made every effort to ensure that the patient care recommended herein, including choice of drugs and drug dosages, is in accord with the accepted standards and practice at the time of publication. However, since research and regulation constantly change clinical standards, the reader is urged to check the product information sheet included in the package of each drug, which includes recommended doses, warnings, and contraindications. This is particularly important with new or infrequently used drugs. Any treatment regimen, particularly one involving medication, involves inherent risk that must be weighed on a case-by-case basis against the benefits anticipated. The reader is cautioned that the purpose of this book is to inform and enlighten; the information contained herein is not intended as, and should not be employed as, a substitute for individual diagnosis and treatment.

Printed in Canada

CONTENTS

Acknowledgments iv

Preface v

1. History of Headache 1

2. Impact of Headache on Society 3

3. Types of Headache 6

4. Causes of Headache 16

5. Danger Signals 24

6. Doctor's Role 25

7. Psychological Factors 27

8. Rebound Headache 31

9. Treatment with Medication 36

10. Treatment without Medication 62

11. Doctor-Patient Relationship 72

12. Emergency Department and Inpatient Treatment . 74

13. Headache in Children 78

14. Hormones and Headache in Women 85

15. Travel, Holidays, and Headache 92

Index 96

ACKNOWLEDGMENTS

We gratefully acknowledge Adrienne Harkavy for her fine touch in editing many drafts of our manuscript. We thank Stephen Mader for his excellent illustrations and Janette Lush and Jennifer Sullivan for their time and efforts in production.

DEDICATION

To our patients who have taught us so much. Don't give up hope.

To my wife and best friend, Karen, for your support and love. To my children, Jason and Lauren, for your patience and understanding. To my parents, Joe and Wilma, for starting it all.

Fred

To my wife, Arja, a very special person, and to our three great children, TJ, Mark, and Sabrina. Thank you all for giving me the time, space, and support to make this a successful project. In honor of my parents, Rose and Jack.

Alan

Since the first edition of *Conquering Headache* was published, our understanding of headache has vastly improved, and during this time, a variety of new treatments have become available or are about to emerge. We wrote this second edition to keep our readers up to date as new developments change the way we think about and treat headache.

Each year, 45 million people in the United States seek medical attention for head pain. Yet headache is an illness largely misunderstood, misdiagnosed, and mistreated. Though the overwhelming majority of headaches are not life threatening, they can be painful and debilitating. For many, headache disrupts daily routines and impairs quality of life.

The vast majority of people with frequent headaches *do not* have tumors, brain aneurysms (weakness in the walls of the blood vessels within the head), allergies, sinus problems, or dental problems. The most common types of headache are migraine, tension-type headache, and to a lesser extent, cluster headache. All these *primary headaches* are *not* due to other medical conditions.

These types of headache are *not* caused by psychological factors. Rather, the primary headaches—migraine, tension-type, and cluster headaches—are the result of biological mechanisms in the brain, blood vessels, and muscles. Can emotional factors play a role? Of course they can, but mostly as headache *triggers* or modulators not as causes.

This book will reveal the truth about headache and will dispel many common myths. Here are the bare facts:

1.   Headache is *not* all in your head.
2.   Allergies do *not* frequently cause headache.
3.   Most headaches are *not* due to sinus problems.
4.   Most headache sufferers *do not* have temporo-mandibular joint (TMJ) syndrome.
5.   More medication for headache is *not* better treatment. In many cases, *less* medication or less potent medications may offer *more relief.*

And this book will point the way to the bottom-line truth about headaches:

6. You *do not* have to learn to live with them!

In this book we will provide you with the information you need to conquer your headaches and improve the quality of your life. You will find the latest information about treatment with medication as well as state-of-the-art updates on nutrition, exercise, sleep habits, behavioral techniques, and pain management. You will also find information about massage, physical therapy, and alternative therapies such as chiropractic, acupuncture, and natural remedies.

In addition, we will give you practical guidelines for medication use—dosages, side effects, and limitations on its use, as well as the tools you need to get your headaches under control and to monitor your progress on paper. The record-keeping systems in this book are the same ones we give to patients in our practice. They include headache calendars to monitor your progress, medication intake and effectiveness, and headache triggers; and—for women—a calendar to monitor menstrual cycles and hormone replacement therapy.

This second edition gives you clear guidelines for dealing with headache in the workplace and in school. Suggestions are provided for children, parents, and teachers. This book *should not be used to self-diagnose or treat.* We encourage you to work closely with your doctor to gain control over your headaches.

Remember that *you* are in charge. The most important factor in conquering your headaches is your willingness to take responsibility, which means you must take an active role in your own recovery. This book alone cannot do it for you, and your doctor cannot do it for you. This book offers information and guidelines to enable you to do the rest. *It will help you learn to control your headaches rather than letting them control you!*

Alan Rapoport, MD, Fred Sheftell, MD.

HISTORY OF HEADACHE

Headache is as old as the human race. Our ancestors believed that headache was visited upon us as punishment for offending the gods or that it occurred when humans became possessed by evil spirits. Not surprisingly, headache remedies were directed toward ridding the body of those demons.

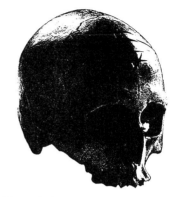

Figure 1–1: Slash marks crisscross a gaping hole in a 12th or 13th century Peruvian girl's skull. The hole shows no signs of bone regrowth, so the girl likely died as a result of her operation. (From the National Museum of Natural History, Washington, DC, catalogue #178473.)

Thus, the earliest neurosurgeons bore holes in the skull through which the headache-causing demons could escape. Skulls with evidence of such surgery were found in Peru and date back to the 14th century (Fig. 1–1).

Hippocrates, a physician who practiced in ancient Greece, noticed that vomiting ended some attacks of head pain, so he prescribed herbs to cause it. He also used another treatment—the application of leeches and bloodletting through small cuts; a practice that persisted through the Middle Ages. The ancient Egyptians wrapped the heads of sufferers in linen along with a clay crocodile holding in its mouth wheat from the gods' storehouse (Fig. 1–2).

By the 17th century, Thomas Willis theorized that headache pain was related to swollen blood vessels in the head. Erasmus Darwin, Charles Darwin's grandfather, further explored these theories. Interestingly, both Charles and Erasmus Darwin suffered from migraine headaches.

Folk remedies such as tying rags around the head or applying tobacco stamps to the head had their advocates, as herbal remedies still do. Heat, cold, acupuncture, chiropractic manipulation, nerve blocks, diets, laser therapies, hyperbaric oxygen, and hysterectomies have also been proposed as headache treatments. There is no shortage of conflicting opinion and information, adding to headache sufferers' confusion about which treatments may or may not help.

It may not be possible to completely cure your headache. The very least you can expect is fewer headaches and better control of the pain.

The remainder of this book will tell you how to take control of your headaches.

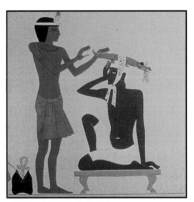

Figure 1–2: Egyptian with clay crocodile with herbs in its mouth placed on his head for headache treatment (courtesy of John Edmeads, MD).

IMPACT OF HEADACHE ON SOCIETY

More patients who visit doctors complain of headache than of any other single ailment. Yet migraine—and headache in general—continues to be underdiagnosed, misdiagnosed, and mistreated. Although medical students learn a great deal about *serious* causes of headache, such as tumors, strokes, aneurysms, and meningitis, they do not learn much about migraine and tension-type headaches, the headaches they will see most frequently in their offices.

Manufacturers of off-the-shelf pain relievers are not permitted by the United States Food and Drug Administration (FDA) to advertise their products for use in migraine headache; they can get around this restriction, however, by suggesting in TV commercials and in advertisements that a headache a doctor might diagnose as a migraine may be due to allergy or sinus problems. The exception is Excedrin.

Headaches, of course, may be due to allergies or sinus problems, but not very often. In addition, many people who worry that their headaches result from psychological factors may seek treatment for sinus and allergy problems, which they would rather believe are the cause of their headaches.

The bulk of nonprescription pain medication is consumed by migraine sufferers and people with chronic daily headache. Headache sufferers are the main purchasers of the 16,000 tons of aspirin, plus much of the acetaminophen (Tylenol), ibuprofen, and sinus medication consumed yearly in the United States. Richard Lipton, MD, estimates that 59% of women and 70% of men with migraine have never been properly diagnosed by a doctor. Lacking a proper diagnosis, these individuals rely on off-the-shelf medicines because they have never received a prescription for a *migraine-specific* medication.

Until the middle of this century, *over-the-counter* meant that you could ask your pharmacist for a bottle of aspirin, and he or she would personally gave it to you—*over the counter*. Today, prescription medications are the only things that pass over the counter; nonprescription medicines are purchased *off the shelf*, most of them through convenience stores, supermarkets, and gas stations (Fig. 2–1).

If nonprescription medication is used improperly, it can have serious consequences. Aspirin can cause peptic ulcer, irritation of the stomach (gastritis), bleeding, bruising, ringing in the ears (tinnitus), and kidney damage; it can also aggravate asthma. Ibuprofen can similarly cause ulcers, bleeding, and kidney damage; and acetaminophen can cause liver damage. Additionally, many sinus and allergy preparations contain ingredients that can raise your blood pressure.

At our Center, we frequently see patients who take 8 to 12 tablets per day of off-the-shelf products. When prescription medications for headache are taken too frequently the problem is even worse. The more frequently a pain medication is taken, the greater the risk of causing chronic, severe headaches that respond poorly to all treatments. So although off-the-shelf pain relievers and other medications targeted for headache are often effective when used properly for occasional headaches, overuse can result in headaches that are harder to treat, more painful, and more constant. These are called *rebound headaches*.

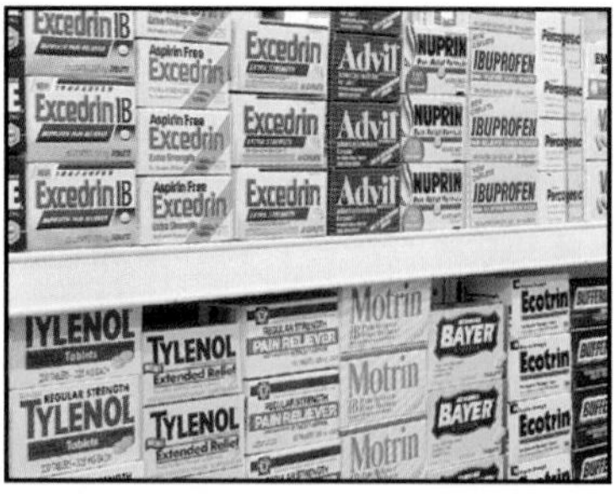

Figure 2–1: Some off-the-shelf medications purchased without supervision.

The impact of headache on our society is enormous: migraine is truly a hidden epidemic. A Canadian survey shows that 92% of migraine sufferers have disability that ranges from diminished ability to function to requiring bed rest! Art created by headache sufferers shows how headache can affect every aspect of their lives. Migraine victims feel cut off from the world around them at work, home, and play.

Headache is the leading cause of absence from the workplace and accounts for loss of some 150 million work days per year in the United States alone; the cost of lost labor hours is estimated to be as high as 17 billion dollars each year. Headache can disrupt every aspect of life outside the workplace and—in an era when some medical costs are not adequately covered by insurance companies—can result in unnecessary medical expense if misdiagnosed or improperly treated.

Society may not understand headache or its impact on those who suffer from it. Workers who telephone their bosses or co-workers to say they cannot come to work because of a headache may be considered malingerers, or worse. Claiming disability due to the flu is more believable. Valerie South, former director of the Canadian Migraine Foundation, points out that "migraine is more than just a 'headache' [it] is a debilitating disorder of the central nervous system."

TYPES OF HEADACHE

Headaches have been classified according to their characteristics to provide a common language for people to use when talking about them.

All headaches can be classified as either *primary* or *secondary*. The secondary headache disorders are those attributable to an underlying medical problem. Serious causes of secondary headache include brain tumors, bleeding in the brain, aneurysms (weakened blood vessel walls), and infections. Less serious causes of secondary headache include dental problems, sinus infections, and allergies. Although TV commercials focus on allergies and sinus problems as causes of headache, the most common types of headaches are primary headaches. These are headaches not attributable to some other medical problem. The primary headache disorders fall into three categories: (1) migraine (2) tension-type headache, and (3) cluster headache.

MIGRAINE

Migraine occurs in more women than men, often causes disability, and affects about 15% of the world's population. Most people with migraine have their first episode of headache between the ages of 6 and 25. The two major categories of migraine are migraine without aura (previously called *common* migraine) and migraine with aura (previously called *classic* migraine). Migraine is usually inherited. Parents with migraine whose children complain of headache should not assume that their children are imitating them. Headache may begin as early as age 2; children of migraine sufferers who complain of headaches should be believed and evaluated by a doctor.

Migraine without Aura

To make a diagnosis of migraine without aura, at least five previous attacks should have occurred; underlying medical conditions or serious causes that could mimic migraine must be ruled out. Attacks may last from 4 to 72 hours, but an average attack usually lasts from 12 to 48 hours.

The diagnosis of migraine without aura requires the presence of two of the four characteristics in group A and one of the three in group B (Table 3–1).

Other symptoms of a migraine attack may include dizziness, frequent urination, diarrhea, sweating, and cold hands and feet. If a fever accompanies your headache, you *must* contact a doctor to rule out a serious infection, such as meningitis. You should, however note that high blood pressure during a migraine attack does not mean you have a persistent high blood pressure problem. To be on the safe side, have your blood pressure checked between headaches to make sure it has returned to normal levels (e.g., 110-120/70-80 mmHg).

Many patients retreat to a dark, quiet room and lie still during attacks; trying to sleep may break a migraine attack.

Table 3–1: Diagnostic Characteristics of Migraine without Aura
Group A (two out of four) Headache on one side of the head Throbbing or pulsating pain Moderate to severe pain that makes it difficult or impossible to function Worsening of pain in response to routine physical activity such as bending over or climbing stairs **Group B (one out of three)** Nausea Vomiting Sensitivity to light and sound

Migraine with Aura

The word *aura* refers to visual symptoms that occur before or at the same time as the headache. Approximately 15% of patients with migraine experience the warning phenomenon of aura. Some patients have aura without headache, which is known as a migraine equivalent. In this case, the headache that follows the aura is similar to that previously described, but less severe.

Aura usually lasts 20 to 30 minutes. The most common type of visual aura shows up as colored spots, flashing bright lights, or multicolored, shimmering, zigzag lines in the shape of a crescent (Fig. 3–1). Other visual disturbances include scotoma (a small, growing black area in the visual field); photopsia (a bright flash of light); loss of vision on one or both sides; tunnel vision, or inability to see words in a particular area when looking at a printed page. Other auras include neurological events that can resemble stroke symptoms, such as weakness or numbness in an arm and/or leg on one side, or difficulty in speaking.

If aura symptoms persist for more than 1 hour, they could be related to a more serious abnormality. In migraine, headache follows the aura in 5 to 60 minutes.

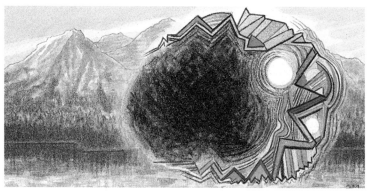

Figure 3–1: Visual aura — changes in vision prior to migraine pain.

MIGRAINE VARIANTS

Migraine variants are seen frequently in some patients.

Exertional Headache

An exertional headache is brought on by exertion of any type, including bending, coughing, sneezing, straining, or exercise. This type of headache should always be brought to a doctor's attention.

Ice-Pick-Like Pains or "Jabs and Jolts"

Also known as "idiopathic (cause unknown) stabbing headache," these headaches are perceived as very sharp, brief, ice-pick-like pains at various locations of the head.

Sex Headache (Coital Headache)

These intense headaches occur primarily in men at the time of orgasm.

Chronic Paroxysmal Hemicrania

This is a rare type of headache disorder that resembles cluster headache. Unlike cluster headache, it occurs more commonly in women than in men and is characterized by 12 or more attacks per day. Always one sided, the pain lasts only 5 to 10 minutes.

All of the above types of headache respond to the non-steroidal anti-inflammatory medication, indomethacin (Indocin), 25 mg, three times per day. Indomethacin is available by prescription.

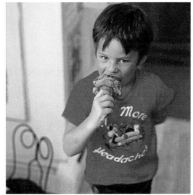

"Ice-Cream" Headache

The official term for this type of headache is "cold stimulus" headache because it occurs between the eyes after eating or drinking something very cold. It

Figure 3–2: A young boy about to experience an "ice-cream" headache.

lasts for fewer than 5 minutes and may be prevented by eating ice cream slowly, in small amounts, and by letting it melt in the mouth before swallowing.

TENSION-TYPE HEADACHE

Tension-type headache is the most common type of headache. Probably 90% or more of the world's population has experienced one from time to time. Many of these headaches are associated with tension in muscles, although in some patients this may not be the case. There is much speculation as to whether tension-type headache and migraine headache are separate disorders. Many headache specialists believe they are caused by similar mechanisms in the brain. Tension-type headaches may be episodic or chronic.

Episodic Tension-Type Headache

Occurring occasionally—once or twice per week, or once per month—these headaches are described as pressing, aching, squeezing, or as a tight band-like feeling that does not throb. It is usually felt on both sides of the head. Unlike migraine, the pain is usually mild or moderate, does not interfere with normal function, and is not aggravated by activity. These headaches are rarely associated with nausea; however, light *or* sound sensitivity may be present, but not both.

Chronic Tension-Type Headache

Symptoms are identical to those of episodic tension-type headache, but they occur more than 15 days per month, often daily. Many patients we see have had these symptoms for months or years when they first visit our office. These patients often develop *chronic daily headache*.

Chronic Daily Headache

At present, there is no official classification for this daily (often constant) headache. Patients say they have pain all the time. Often they add that it waxes and wanes throughout the day. It wears them down. Occasionally, the pain becomes sufficiently severe that it interferes with their ability to function. This type of headache clearly resembles migraine. Some experts believe these patients have *transformed migraine*, which starts in the teens with occasional migraine, and *transforms* to daily, dull-to-moderate pain (tension-type headache) by the time they are in their 30s and 40s. Eighty percent of people with chronic daily headache take pain relievers or other acute care medications on a daily basis. As a result, this can lead to *rebound* headache, which is worse and more constant (see Chapter 8).

CLUSTER HEADACHE

Cluster headache is probably the most dramatic of all the headache types. The pain occurs exclusively on one side of the head, in and around the eye and temple. In contrast to typical throbbing migraine pain, cluster pain is more steady, boring, and relentless.

Patients describe pain as intense pressure behind the eye that feels as though it is pushing the eye forward. Some patients describe the feeling as one which makes them want to pluck out the painful eye. Others describe it as a red-hot poker being thrust into the eye with immense force and then twirled. Drooping of the eyelid, constriction of the pupil, redness and tearing of the eye, followed by a stuffed then running nostril, may accompany the headache, occurring on the same side of the head as the pain. It may last anywhere from 20 minutes to 3 hours, with an average duration of 45 to 90 minutes.

Attacks may occur several times per day with an average of one to three attacks in a 24-hour period. Cluster headaches often occur at the same time of the day or night, usually after work. Most characteristically, these headaches awaken the sufferer 90 minutes after falling asleep.

In contrast to migraine, which affects one in five women and occurs three times more frequently in women than in men, cluster headaches occur five times as often in men and affect only 0.1% of the population. A family history of cluster headache is much less common than migraine. The typical male sufferer is 35 years old, a little taller than average, and may have hazel-colored eyes, along with deep lines around the forehead, mouth, and chin.

Cluster pain is so excruciating that it brings even the strongest of men literally to their knees. It is no wonder that cluster headache has been termed "suicide headache." Rather than retreating to a dark, quiet room as do migraine sufferers, cluster patients cannot sit or lie still. Rather, they pace, rock, and drive their fists into the painful eye. Some patients may even show unusual behavior, such as hitting themselves in the head, banging their heads against the wall, or engaging in intense physical activity such as push-ups or running.

The word "cluster" describes the time pattern of these headaches, which occur in cluster periods of about 6 to 8 weeks per year. Patients are free of headache between cluster periods. Alcohol is the most common trigger, but only during the cluster period. Actively drinking alcoholics may stop drinking completely until the cluster period has passed. Cluster headache occurs in two patterns: episodic and chronic.

Episodic Cluster Headache

In the more common episodic variety of cluster headache, patients experience a 6-week cluster period once per year. Cluster periods may occur every 1 to 2 years, or only once in a lifetime. Symptoms may mislead doctors to incorrect diagnoses and treatments such as sinus headaches which may be inappropriately treated with a variety of sinus medications and surgery. They may also be mistaken for dental problems or temporomandibular joint (TMJ) dysfunction (see page 15).

Chronic Cluster Headache

About 10% of all patients suffering from cluster headaches have them on a daily, or almost-daily, basis for years. Fortunately, we now have effective treatments for cluster headaches.

OTHER HEADACHE TYPES

Post-Traumatic Headache

Post-traumatic headaches sometimes follow injury to the head or neck and may even develop after what seems to be only a minor injury. These headaches usually occur on both sides of the head; they are constant and mild to moderate in intensity; and they can continue for months. Sometimes, they become severe, or even incapacitating and resemble migraine. Patients with post-traumatic headache may be thought to be exaggerating their pain or malingering, but in our experience, these patients have a debilitating disorder that may destroy the fabric of their lives which may seriously impair their ability to function.

Some patients with post-traumatic headache also develop the post-head trauma syndrome and experience impaired concentration, memory, and sleep, as well as irritability, decreased energy and interests, personality changes, and decreased ability to handle even simple tasks.

Although scans of the brain or the cervical spine fail to reveal abnormalities, the injury may have caused microscopic tearing and damage to nerve fibers in the brain and brain stem. The damage may disrupt the delicate balance of the chemical messengers that control pain. Many patients develop post-traumatic headache as a result of a "whiplash" (or neck injury) after a rear-end car accident. The degree of head trauma does not necessarily correlate with the degree of pain intensity or disability. Pre-existing migraine or tension-type headache may worsen after this kind of injury.

Sinus Headache

Sinus problems rarely cause chronic headaches. Sinus headaches are due to inflammation of the mucous membranes lining the sinuses in the head. Blockage of the sinus drainage system may cause infection and these infections are classified as acute or chronic. Headache caused by acute sinusitis may be felt in the cheeks, below, above, or behind the eyes, or it may be *referred* to other areas such as the teeth or the top of the head.

Acute sinusitis is generally associated with fever, red, hot skin over the sinus, and a yellow-green discharge from the nostrils and back of the throat. Any headache associated with fever or infection *must* be treated immediately.

Chronic, low-grade inflammation of any of the sinuses in the head may cause headache. The pain patterns are similar to those in acute sinusitis but of lesser intensity and not usually associated with fever. Depending on the sinuses involved, pain may be increased by shaking the head or by lying in certain positions that decrease the ability of the sinuses to drain. A severe sinus problem may trigger a migraine attack.

Allergy Headache

Commercials and advertisements to the contrary, most headaches are not due to allergies. Allergy to pollen and grasses, and hay fever can, however, cause sinus pain and headache.

Eye-Related Headache

Eye strain is not a common cause of chronic or recurrent headache. Headaches that *are* due to eye strain are generally mild and are felt in the forehead or in the eyes themselves. The pain is absent on awakening and worsens when the eyes are used for prolonged periods.

Glaucoma (increased pressure within the eye) may cause a headache that mimics a bad migraine or tension-type headache or it may cause severe pain in and around the eye or in the forehead. If you notice changes in your vision accompanied by pain and other symptoms, consult an eye doctor at once.

Temporomandibular Joint Dysfunction (TMD)

The temporomandibular joint (TMJ) is located just in front of the ear, where the jaw meets the skull. TMJ problems may cause ear or jaw pain, ringing in the ears, or pain (headache) in the area where the hinges of the jaw meet the upper face.

Many patients have been misdiagnosed as having TMJ problems and have undergone major surgical reconstruction of the joint without experiencing any relief of their pain. Most "TMJ headaches" are actually migraine or tension-type headaches.

Trigeminal Neuralgia

Trigeminal neuralgia is a piercing, sudden, severe pain lasting 1 to 4 minutes, confined to the cheek or jaw on one side. This type of pain is triggered by talking, chewing, exposure to wind, or even by touching the face.

Spinal Tap Headache

Spinal tap headache occurs 12 to 48 hours after a diagnostic spinal tap in which fluid is removed from the spinal column. It is a diffuse, steady pain accompanied by nausea. It gets worse on standing and disappears on lying down. The headache occurs because fluid leaks from the spinal column at the spot where the needle made its puncture. The treatment is to drink sufficient fluids and to lie absolutely flat for 2 days. This type of headache disappears slowly. In severe cases, a minor procedure called an epidural blood patch is performed to seal the hole and prevent further leakage of spinal fluid.

CAUSES OF HEADACHE

Our patients frequently ask us, "What causes my headaches?" Another frequently asked question is, "If all my tests are normal, and nothing's *seriously* wrong, why do I get headaches?"

Understandably, patients with unexplained symptoms fear the worst, and when most causes of headache have been ruled out, they may fall back on media-driven explanations that attribute headache to sinus, allergy, and jaw problems. It is not surprising when test results come back normal that many patients fear their headaches are not "real," but rather the result of a psychological process. This, of course, is not usually the case.

Unfortunately, there are no *biologic* markers or accurate tests to confirm the diagnosis of the most common headache disorders. Diagnosis of headache is based on medical history, neurological and physical examination, and appropriate tests. Most causes of headache probably do not show up on routine tests because we do not yet have the specific means to measure biochemical and electrical changes in the brain, the blood vessels, and the muscles.

CAUSES OF MIGRAINE

A tendency to develop migraine is inherited; up to 90% of people with migraine have a close relative who gets them, too. Your family history can give your doctor important information that may suggest migraine as a diagnosis. Some studies show that if one parent has migraine, each child has a 40% chance of developing it; if both parents have migraine, each child has a 75% chance.

Four main theories about the cause of migraine have been proposed. The theories center on the following: (1) the brain (the central theory); (2) the blood vessels (the vascular theory); (3) inflammation (the neurogenic inflammation theory, which involves the trigeminovascular system), (Fig. 4–1); and (4) a combination of these factors (the unifying theory), which helps to pull the three interrelated theories together.

The Brain: Central Theory

K.M.A. Welch, MD, a neurologist in Detroit has observed that magnesium levels in the brain are low in migraine patients. His theory holds that low magnesium levels may trigger abnormal brain electrical activity that starts in the back of the brain during the aura phase and spreads forward. A second part of the central theory focuses on biochemical changes that occur in the brain stem (see Fig. 4–1), where the nerves rely on a chemical called serotonin. Neil Raskin, MD, of San Francisco, believes that headache results from a disturbance of serotonin activity in the midbrain, which is part of the brain stem. The fact that several effective antimigraine drugs affect serotonin receptors suggests that this may be the case.

The Blood Vessels: Vascular Theory

In the 17th century Sir Thomas Willis proposed that migraine was caused by changes in blood vessel activity, a theory updated at The New York Hospital during the 1930s by Harold Wolff, MD, and John Graham, MD. The fact that ergotamine tartrate, given intravenously, noticeably decreases the painful throbbing and pulse of swollen arteries in the scalp supports this theory. It is also possible that platelets—serotonin-containing blood cells involved in clotting—are abnormal in migraine sufferers. This is why some doctors believe that small, daily doses of aspirin, which reduce the platelets' ability to clump, may be helpful in reducing the frequency of mild migraine.

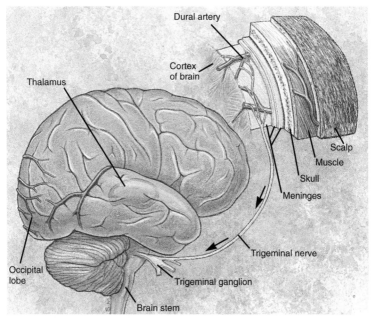

Figure 4–1: Anatomy of brain and scalp — showing trigeminovascular system.

The Trigeminovascular System: Neurogenic Inflammation Theory

Michael Moskowitz, MD, a headache researcher from Boston, has shown that the trigeminovascular system of the brain is the key to migraine pain. This system involves one of the twelve cranial nerves—the trigeminal (or 5th cranial nerve)—and its interface with the arteries in the covering of brain (the meninges). Chemicals released from the ends of the trigeminal nerve cause inflammation to occur around blood vessels. Many medicines effective in treating migraine—including the "triptans" and ergotamines (see Chapter 9)—act at the interface of the trigeminal nerve endings and the vascular system in the meninges.

Unifying Theory

Jim Lance, MD, of Sydney, Australia believes that migraine represents a succession of events that begins in one area of the brain as an electrical change and causes alterations in another area of the brain and the trigeminovascular system. These changes trigger biochemical events in the brain that result in clumping of platelets; alterations in blood vessel size; and release of pain-producing substances, some of which are related to serotonin.

Nat Blau, MD, of London, England, points out that even patients who do not experience a visual aura often have a set of symptoms—a *prodrome*—that may occur hours before migraine pain begins. Prodrome symptoms include fatigue, a feeling of great energy or exhilaration, changes in activity level, yawning, or changes in appetite and sleep patterns. All these symptoms originate deep in the brain, suggesting that the migraine process begins there.

MIGRAINE TRIGGERS

Many migraine patients are unusually sensitive to internal (within the body) and external (outside the body) environmental change (Table 4–1). A variety of factors can trigger an explosive migraine attack. The menstrual cycle is clearly a major trigger in the great majority of women; a second trigger is food. Although alcoholic beverages are common triggers, red wine and beer are the drinks most frequently mentioned by patients. The dark-colored alcohols (scotch, bourbon, dark rum, and red wine) appear more likely to trigger migraine attacks than the light-colored ones (gin, vodka, white rum, and white wine). Many foods (Table 4–2), particularly those that contain tyramine, trigger migraine.

Monosodium glutamate (MSG), an ingredient added to a wide variety of prepared foods, can trigger migraine. Read food labels carefully! Look for MSG and for hydrolyzed fat

Table 4-1: Environmental Triggers of Migraine

Internal
  Chronic fatigue, too little sleep
  Emotional stress, let-down after stress
  Hormonal fluctuations (menstrual cycle)
External
  Weather and seasonal change
  Travel through time zones (see Chapter 15)
  Altitude
  Skipping or delaying meals
  Sensory stimuli
    Flickering or bright lights, sunlight
    Odors, including perfume, chemicals, cigarette smoke
    Heat, loud noises
  Medications (see Chapter 8)
    Nitroglycerin
    Tetracycline (an antibiotic)
    High doses of vitamin A
    Some antidepressant medications (SSRIs)
    Some blood pressure medications

or hydrolyzed protein. Both Nutrasweet, the food ingredient, and Equal, the sugar substitute, contain aspartame, and both have been associated with headache in susceptible individuals.

Since caffeine may help constrict blood vessels during a migraine attack, it is used in combination products to increase pain relief (e.g., Excedrin is a combination of aspirin, acetaminophen, and caffeine); habitual consumption of too much caffeine, however, can make headaches worse.

Table 4-2: Dietary Triggers

Chocolate	Onions	Nutrasweet, Equal (aspartame)
Nuts	Pizza	Canned figs
Peanut butter	Avocado	Aged cheese
Bananas	Processed meats	Caffeine (see Table 4-3)
Alcoholic beverages	Hot dogs, pepperoni	
Red wine	Sausages, bacon, ham	
Others	Bologna, salami	
	Pickled/fermented foods	
	Yogurt	
	Sour cream	

Table 4–3: Caffeine Content of Common Foods and Drugs

Product	Example	Caffeine Content (mg)
Cocoa and chocolate	Chocolate candy bar	25
	Cocoa beverage (6 oz mixture)	10
Coffee	Decaffeinated (5 oz)	2
	Drip (5 oz)	146
	Instant, regular (5 oz)	53
	Percolated (5 oz)	110
Off-the-shelf drugs	Anacin	32
	Extra-Strength Excedrin	65
	No-Doz tablets	100-200
	Vanquish	33
	Vivarin tablets	200
Prescription drugs	Darvon Compound-65	32.4
	Esgic	40
	Fioricet	40
	Fiorinal	40
Soft drinks (12 oz)	7-Up/Diet 7-Up	0
	Coca-Cola	34
	Diet Pepsi	34
	Dr. Pepper	38
Tea	3-minute brew (5 oz)	22-46

But how much caffeine is too much? Some patients are sensitive to the small amount of caffeine in one 5-ounce cup of brewed coffee (approximately 100 mg). Many patients who complain of headaches on Saturday or Sunday mornings take less caffeine on weekends than during the week or they sleep later, thus drinking their coffee later in the morning. Headaches that occur under these circumstances could be due to caffeine withdrawal and are more likely to occur in people who are accustomed to drinking more than 300 mg of caffeine per day. At 500 mg per day or above, caffeinism, with symptoms that include disturbed sleep, anxiety, nervousness, and increased irritability, may occur. Table 4–3 lists the caffeine content of various products.

Stress and Migraine
Although stress is high on the list of migraine triggers, if you are not biologically predisposed to migraine, stress will not cause you to get a headache. Migraine is, however, likely to occur during let-down periods, such as after the stress has come and gone, or during a period of unwinding or relaxing. This may explain why many patients have migraine attacks on weekends or on vacations.

CAUSES OF TENSION-TYPE HEADACHE

Early theories of tension-type headache attributed the pain to contraction of muscles around the head and neck, which explains why this type of headache was originally termed muscle contraction headache. It is true, however, that tension-type headache may occur in people who—for one reason or another—unconsciously tighten up the muscles around the head and neck. Poor posture, tense jaw, temporomandibular joint problems, arthritis, disc disease in the neck, and occupational factors, such as sitting for long periods at computer terminals, typing, or cradling the phone between the ear and shoulder may all be associated with tension-type headache.

It is easy to see how tight muscles could be related to tension-type headache, but factors within the brain may be involved as well.

Possible Connections between Tension-Type Headache and Migraine
Since some of the symptoms of tension-type headache and migraine overlap, and since many people suffer from both types of headache, some headache specialists believe that

these two conditions are related. Many patients may develop an acute tension-type headache that over a period of hours may evolve into a clear-cut migraine. It is not surprising that one group of headache specialists believes that headaches represent a *continuum* that includes tension-type headache and migraine, which share similar underlying mechanisms and that the other group considers the two headache types to be completely *distinct* disorders.

Depression and anxiety that may be associated with chronic daily headache should be addressed as part of a patient's whole headache picture.

CAUSES OF CLUSTER HEADACHE

The causes of cluster headache are complex. According to Lee Kudrow, MD, of Los Angeles, a current theory proposes that a tiny nerve bundle that regulates body rhythms deep within the brain is responsible for bringing on cluster headaches with clock-like regularity. Lithium carbonate has provided effective treatment for some patients, perhaps because it is believed to regulate the hypothalamus, which houses the biological clock.

CONCLUSION

Further clarification of the biological mechanisms responsible for headache will help doctors understand more about headache and will yield more specific treatments that clinicians can offer to their patients.

CHAPTER 5

DANGER SIGNALS

More than 95% of headaches are primary headaches that are not caused by serious underlying medical conditions. You should, however, be aware of the *red flags* or *danger signals* listed below, because these are signs that you should seek medical attention. If you:

1. rarely get headaches and suddenly develop a *severe* one.
2. often get headaches and develop a new, *severe* type or one that comes on suddenly and remains.
3. develop the *worst headache* you have ever had.
4. develop a headache that gradually worsens over a period of days or weeks (it could be that a tumor, an infection, or an aneurysm [bulging blood vessel] is pressing on pain-sensitive structures).
5. get headaches when you exercise, cough, sneeze, or bend over (they could be migraine or benign exertional headaches, but you may have something more serious).
6. get a "bug" or virus, and you develop a severe headache accompanied by nausea and vomiting and a neck so stiff that you cannot put your chin on your chest without pain, you *must* seek medical attention *right away* to rule out meningitis.
7. get a headache accompanied by any of the following neurological symptoms—impaired speech, trouble with coordination, weakness or numbness in any extremity, or on one side of the body, drowsiness, inability to stay awake, confusion, or a change in personality, consult a doctor.

In general, a new onset headache in someone who does not usually get headaches, who gets a headache more severe than usual, who experiences a significant change in a typical headache or a headache that escalates in severity more rapidly than usual or steadily over many days should be evaluated medically as soon as possible.

CHAPTER 6

THE DOCTOR'S ROLE

When you visit your own physician, a neurologist, or a headache specialist, you will be questioned about your headaches. The doctor will ask about each type of headache you get, e.g., when did it start; how frequently do you get this type; how long does it last; where is the pain located, and how severe is it; are there other symptoms associated with it; what brings it on (triggers it); and what makes it better?

Your doctor will then do a neurological examination and evaluate your mental alertness, cranial nerve function, including vision and hearing, strength, coordination and gait, reflexes, and ability to perceive different sensations. In addition, your blood pressure, pulse, and the state of the arteries in your head and neck will be noted.

Although the histories of migraine sufferers are dramatic, they usually turn out to have normal neurological examinations.

Even if your examination is normal, your doctor may order blood tests to check for infection and inflammation, metabolic problems, liver or thyroid dysfunction, and perhaps for Lyme disease, anemia, and other conditions that might contribute to your headaches. Do not be surprised if your doctor sends you for a computed tomography (CT) or a magnetic resonance imaging (MRI) scan of your head since this is the best way to rule out serious structural problems in the brain. Both CT and MRI scans are painless. CT scans involve use of x-rays; an iodine-containing dye may be injected into an arm vein to increase the contrast of the images. Be sure to tell your doctor if you are allergic to iodine. MRI scans do not use x-rays but are done in a strong magnetic field. Dye may be injected into an arm vein. Most MRI machines resemble a small tunnel, open at both ends. MRI scans usually cost 40–100% more than CT scans, but they provide more detailed information. Pregnant women should not have either scan, but an MRI is preferable to a CT scan when imaging is necessary.

A spinal tap (lumbar puncture) may be indicated, if your headaches are severe or are associated with stiff neck, fever, vomiting, and signs of increased pressure in the brain. The most important abnormal findings from a spinal tap are evidence of bleeding, infection, or increased pressure. Patients are often told to lie flat for several hours after a spinal tap to avoid an increase in headache pain. An electroencephalogram (EEG) can be useful when evaluating headache patients whose histories include fainting, loss of consciousness, head trauma, or dizziness.

The most important part of your evaluation is the *history* your doctor obtains from you. It alone can point to an accurate tentative diagnosis that can be confirmed by appropriate examination and testing.

Be sure to tell your doctor the impact your headaches have on your life.

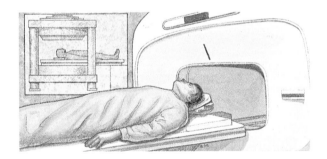

Figure 6–1: Magnetic resonance imaging (MRI) scan.

CHAPTER 7

PSYCHOLOGICAL FACTORS

Until recently, the biologic basis of head pain was poorly understood. This may be why headache is not always considered a legitimate complaint and why some patients with headache are not taken seriously. We still do not have all the answers, but we do know that headache has a firm basis in the biology of the brain.

Although psychological factors, such as personality style and stress, can influence headache, they rarely cause it. All medical disorders, however, *are* affected by psychological factors. We cannot completely separate our minds from our bodies.

Psychological factors, the least common cause of headache, fall into three categories: (1) those that cause it; (2) those that contribute to it; and (3) those that coexist with it.

PSYCHOLOGICAL FACTORS THAT CAUSE HEADACHE

Psychogenic

The term psychogenic suggests that the pain is either not real or that it is somehow different from real pain.

Malingering

Malingering is the intentional production of false symptoms, in other words, conscious lying or faking. It may occur when someone is trying to avoid situations such as school, work, jail, or combat duty. However, we rarely see malingerers, even among patients whose head pain results from trauma.

Migraine Personality

The term migraine personality has generated much confusion. The origin of the term is attributed to Harold Wolff, MD, a neurologist who was working at the New York Hospital in the early 1960s and noticed that a large percentage of his migraine patients seemed to have strikingly similar personality characteristics. Today, however, we know that the personalities of migraine sufferers differ very little from those of the rest of the population.

PSYCHOLOGICAL FACTORS THAT CONTRIBUTE TO HEADACHE

We believe that the common primary headache is biologic in origin and genetically determined. If, however, one has the biologic vulnerability to develop headache, behavioral changes and stress may *trigger* one.

Stress

The body is subject to stress when called upon to react to changes in the environment. When stress is overwhelming or constant, physical or emotional symptoms may occur. Any of the following may be stressful: difficulties at the workplace, marital problems, financial problems, difficulty in school, and caring for a sick relative. Stress is not always negative. Positive events such as purchasing a house, getting married, having a child, moving, or changing jobs can be stressful, too.

Migraine patients often do well when they are going at full speed. They may, however, develop migraine after the stress has been resolved and they begin to relax, which explains why some patients may experience attacks on weekends and during vacations. Patients suffering from cluster headaches tend to get their headaches during the letdown after work, when they are relaxing after a hard day. This is not a psychological phenomenon, but one which can be explained by changes in brain chemistry.

PSYCHIATRIC DISORDERS THAT COEXIST WITH HEADACHE (COMORBIDITY)

Migraine and related disorders do not protect an individual from developing psychiatric problems or other physical problems. The incidence of depression, anxiety disorders such as panic attacks, phobias, and sleep disorders is higher in patients with migraine and chronic daily headache. Although the exact relationship between head pain, anxiety, sleep disorders, and depression is not completely understood, we do know that serotonin, a chemical that occurs naturally in the

---

Table 7-1: Common Symptoms of Depression and Anxiety

Depression
- Depressed mood
- Decreased ability to experience pleasure and decreased interests
- Significant changes in weight
- Persistent difficulty in falling asleep or staying asleep
- Sleeping too much
- Others have observed that you are markedly slowed down or agitated
- Decreased energy or increased fatigue
- Feelings of worthlessness, guilt, decreased concentration, and inability to make even simple decisions
- Recurrent thoughts of death

Anxiety
- Shortness of breath or a feeling of smothering
- Dizziness or feelings of unsteadiness
- Palpitations or rapid heart beat
- Trembling or shaking
- Sweating
- Choking or trouble swallowing
- Nausea or abdominal distress
- A feeling that you are not real or that your environment is somehow not real or changed
- Numbness or tingling sensations
- Chills or flushing
- Chest pain
- Fear of dying
- Fear of going crazy or doing something that you cannot control

brain, plays a role. The "serotonin connection" suggests that all these disorders share an underlying biological cause.

In the absence of physical findings, it is easy to understand that anyone with chronic pain can become depressed. Some still view psychiatric disorders as the primary causes of chronic pain. Table 7–1 lists some common symptoms of depression and anxiety disorders. If you experience symptoms of anxiety or depression, you may want to consider the possibility that you have a treatable psychological problem.

Head pain is depressed patients' most frequent physical complaint. Patients with chronic daily headache may also have depressive symptoms that include difficulty sleeping, decreased interest in everything they formerly enjoyed, decreased energy, and decreased concentration. If depression or anxiety coexist with your headache disorder, it is difficult to treat one without addressing the other. Do not be upset if your doctor suggests that you may be anxious or depressed. He or she is trying to manage all the factors that may contribute to your headache.

CONCLUSION

Psychological factors may contribute to your headaches, but they are rarely the cause. A variety of psychological tests may help to identify depression and anxiety. Other disorders such as alcoholism and other forms of substance abuse must be identified as well. Although many headache patients may overuse medication, they are not substance abusers, but are using these substances in an effort to remain functional.

CHAPTER 8

REBOUND HEADACHE

Headaches can be made worse by overuse of off-the-shelf and prescription pain relievers such as aspirin and acetaminophen, barbiturates, caffeine, and ergotamine tartrate. Overuse can result in analgesic rebound headache. In addition, some medications prescribed for medical conditions other than headache may worsen or produce headache.

ANALGESIC REBOUND HEADACHE

Increasing your consumption of pain medication not only fails to relieve headache, it may perpetuate and intensify it, resulting in analgesic rebound headache. Most headache specialists agree that taking pain medications three or more days in a week, greatly increases the risk of developing rebound headache. What's more, taking off-the-shelf medications—even as few as 2 to 4 tablets every day—can produce it. Many patients who develop rebound headache take more than one kind of pain reliever. Headache medicines are often a combination of products (see Chapter 9) that include a variety of pain relievers, caffeine, and other substances that affect blood vessels. Although it is not known exactly which medications produce this syndrome, it is possible that even aspirin and acetaminophen—alone or in combination, with or without caffeine—can cause it. The nonsteroidal anti-inflammatory medications might also cause rebound headache. Two of the more common ingredients related to rebound headache are butalbital, which is in Fiorinal, Fioricet, Phrenilin, and Esgic, and codeine, which is in Fiorinal with codeine, Fioricet with codeine, Tylenol with codeine, and similar preparations, sold under various brand and generic names. Sedatives and tranquilizers may also cause rebound headache. Additionally, overuse of these medications tends to reduce the usual effectiveness of daily preventive medications, relaxation techniques, and biofeedback training. Daily caffeine intake from beverages and mixed analgesics may also contribute to your headache problem (see page 33).

So how does overuse of pain medications come about? Let's say you often wake up in the morning with a mild headache that you are afraid will get worse. So, you take a small dose of off-the-shelf pain reliever. You might, just to be on the "safe" side, take a dose every morning. Before long, you might be taking 2 pills every 4 hours—or 6 to 12 tablets a day. Then, over time, your headaches seem to get worse, which leads you to increase the number of pills you take. Before you know it, you are taking large amounts of medication, and instead of feeling better, you feel worse.

How to Recognize Rebound Headache

A typical rebound headache lasts between 4 and 24 hours. The pain is mild to moderate, dull, nonthrobbing, and steady. It can occur in any part of the head or all over the head, and is usually felt on both sides of the head rather than on one side. In most cases, patients do not experience migraine-type symptoms, such as throbbing, nausea, increased sensitivity to light and sound, or pain worsening with mild exertion. Sometimes, however, the pain can intensify into a severe migraine episode.

Patients may become anxious and depressed, may have difficulty falling asleep or, even more commonly, may awaken early and be unable to get back to sleep. They may also be irritable, have trouble concentrating, and they may experience other neurological and psychological symptoms.

Patients with analgesic rebound who have tried to stop overusing pain relievers know that their headaches will worsen before they get better. Their headaches may intensify within 4 to 6 hours after stopping the medication, becoming most intense within 1 to 2 days. This withdrawal period may last for 2 to 3 weeks. In some cases, the symptoms can be relieved by

Midrin, nonsteroidal anti-inflammatory medications, antinausea medications, or tranquilizers.

After gradually stopping their use of analgesics, most patients notice an improvement in their headache symptoms and in their general sense of well-being within 2 to 3 months. They note that their headaches are less frequent and less severe. They feel better, sleep better, and are less depressed, and they worry less about getting headaches.

Once overuse of pain relievers is under control, patients find that they respond to daily preventive medications, such as beta-blockers, calcium blockers, and antidepressants. None of these would be effective during analgesic rebound headache.

ERGOTAMINE REBOUND HEADACHE

Although ergotamine tartrate is effective in relieving acute migraine, its overuse results in an ergotamine rebound syndrome. Because it relieves migraine headache quickly, patients with rebound may use ergotamine for each headache, even mild ones, and they soon find that their ergotamine-responsive headaches occur more frequently.

CAFFEINE REBOUND HEADACHE

Many headache preparations contain caffeine, a blood vessel constrictor which, when combined with analgesics, boosts pain relief. Caffeine can produce headache both when overused on a regular basis and when it is stopped abruptly (see Chapter 4).

At our Center, patients are questioned carefully about their caffeine intake. If it is high—over 250 mg per day, equivalent to 2½ cups of coffee, we ask them to reduce their coffee consumption slowly by one cup per week, over a period of 2 to 3 weeks, to avoid worsening headaches. Patients who abstain from caffeine for a month can resume drinking one cup of regular coffee per day and as much decaffeinated coffee as they like.

TREATMENT OF REBOUND SYNDROMES

Treatment of rebound syndromes begins with an assessment and a prescription for a behavioral wellness program. Patients should be given a detailed explanation of the syndrome as well as help in withdrawing from overused medications and tips on avoiding the syndrome in the future. Biofeedback training and relaxation techniques can be helpful, particularly when incorporated in a comprehensive behavioral program.

The key to treatment is to discontinue the overused drug and to break the cycle of daily headache. Off-the-shelf medication can be withdrawn gradually over a few days, but prescription medications should be discontinued more slowly. Medications such as opiates, butalbital-containing medications (such as Fiorinal), and caffeine-containing medications should be reduced over a period of several weeks. Patients using large amounts of opiates or ergotamines for a significant period of time often require hospitalization, enabling them to receive effective doses of medication to prevent a severe worsening of headache and other symptoms as they withdraw from the offending medication. Outpatients should be seen frequently in the office, until withdrawal has been completed.

The most effective in-hospital treatment is the administration of intravenous dihydroergotamine (D.H.E. 45), to which intravenous steroids may be added. After detoxification is complete, appropriate combinations of preventive medication can be prescribed.

The follow-up behavioral wellness program should include self-help techniques, dietary instruction, an exercise and fitness program, and appropriate counseling.

NONHEADACHE DRUGS THAT MAY CAUSE HEADACHE

Some nonheadache medications can cause headache (Table 8–1). Indomethacin (Indocin), a potent nonsteroidal anti-inflammatory medication, is very effective in some headache syndromes. Some patients who take it for nonheadache reasons may develop excruciating headaches which often send them to an emergency room for evaluation. Once a serious problem has been ruled out and indomethacin discontinued, the headache promptly resolves.

Nifedipine (Procardia), an effective calcium channel blocker used to treat high blood pressure by dilating blood vessels, may induce a severe, throbbing headache—even in nonheadache patients. A similar headache may occur in patients who take nitroglycerin for chest pain.

TREATMENT WITH MEDICATION

At The New England Center for Headache, in Stamford, Connecticut, patients are treated with both pharmacologic and nonpharmacologic methods (as described in Chapter 10). Our philosophy is to use as few medications as possible, at the smallest doses possible, for the shortest possible period of time. We start with low doses of the milder medications and increase dosage and potency as necessary.

Overuse of medication designed to treat acute headache can lead to rebound syndromes and dependency. Our major concern is with the number of days per week on which patients take pain relievers, rather than the amount taken on any given day. We limit use of medication to 3 days per week, since even small amounts taken daily may induce analgesic rebound headache.

Each patient's medication program is based on the individual's needs. All patients, however, must accurately record how they use medication on a daily basis on a headache calendar (see Fig. 10–1a).

Headache medication falls into three categories, as follows:

1. Symptomatic treatment: medications in this category are directed at *symptoms* such as pain, nausea, or vomiting; they may also help patients to relax and possibly sleep.
2. Specific treatment: medications in this category *interfere* with the *process* that causes the headache to stop pain and its associated symptoms, nausea, vomiting, or sensitivity to light and sound.
3. Preventive (prophylactic) treatment: medications in this category are taken daily to prevent frequently occurring headache. They may also be prescribed for patients who experience 3 to 4 or more severe migraine attacks per month and who have not experienced adequate relief from specific medication. The beneficial effects of these medications may not be evident for some weeks. Patients

should not discontinue such medications without medical advice, since stopping them abruptly could result in serious side effects.

Warning: All medications have side effects. Patients should understand the desired effects of medications, how they work, and the side effects that may occur. Whenever we prescribe medication, we give our patients a list of side effects so that they can watch out for them. To avoid side effects, we start medication at low doses and build up slowly to the optimal dose.

EARLY TREATMENT OF HEADACHE ATTACKS

The earlier a headache is "caught" and treated, the greater the likelihood that it can be relieved with milder medication. Patients who wait many hours into the course of a headache before beginning treatment may find that stronger medications are required or that all medications are less effective. The trick is *not* to treat mild headaches with medication—these tend to go away on their own. The best time to take medication is when a headache begins to *worsen*—before it sets in and becomes more difficult to treat. Since medications alone are not the whole answer, we recommend alternative forms of therapy, such as the application of a cold pack to the temples, forehead, eyes, or nape of the neck. Taking a warm or hot shower sometimes works, as does resting in a comfortable position in a quiet, dark area. All these techniques may help increase the effectiveness of medication.

TREATMENT OF ACUTE TENSION-TYPE HEADACHE

Our patients learn to differentiate between an acute tension-type headache and a more significant migraine attack. At the beginning of an attack, it may, however, be difficult for some patients to tell the difference. Simple, single-ingredient pain medications such as aspirin, acetaminophen, and nonsteroidal anti-inflammatory agents (such as ibuprofen, ketoprofen, and

Table 9–1: Off-the-Shelf Simple Analgesics

	Ingredients		
	Aspirin (mg)	Acetaminophen (mg)	Other (mg)
Advil			ibuprofen 200
Aleve			naproxen sodium 220
Anacin III		325	
Anacin III (maximum strength)		500	
Aspirin	325		
Bayer Aspirin	325		
Bayer Aspirin (8-hr time release)	625		
Bayer Aspirin (maximum)	500		
Bayer Aspirin (therapy)	325		
Datril E.S.		500	
Ecotrin (enteric-coated)	325		
Ecotrin maximum strength (enteric-coated)	500		
Empirin	325		
Ibuprofen			ibuprofen 200
Medipren			ibuprofen 200
Motrin IB			ibuprofen 200
Nuprin			ibuprofen 200
Panadol		500	
Tylenol		325	
Tylenol (extra-strength)		500	

naproxen) are sufficient for most tension-type headaches. More severe attacks usually respond to combination medications, which include caffeine and barbiturates, isomethoptene (Midrin), and occasionally opiates (narcotics), such as codeine. Patients with a tension-type headache do not usually experience nausea, but antinausea medications may be useful if gastrointestinal effects accompany the headache. Your physician's choice of medication will take into account such factors as your health, your medical and family history, and other prescription and nonprescription drugs you may be taking.

Treatment Plan
Option 1:

Begin with two regular strength aspirin tablets or a non-steroidal anti-inflammatory drug (NSAID), such as ibuprofen (Motrin IB, Advil, Nuprin, etc.); naproxen sodium, (Aleve); or ketoprofen (Orudis KT). If these irritate your stomach or cause you to bruise easily, start instead with two extra-strength acetaminophen (Tylenol) tablets (Table 9–1).

Side effects. Aspirin and the NSAIDs can interfere with blood clotting, which may cause you to bruise more easily (you may notice black-and-blue marks on your body), or for cuts or gums to bleed more easily when you brush or floss. Be sure to get in touch with your doctor if you notice such signs. Acetaminophen-containing preparations do not interfere with blood clotting, but if taken in sufficient quantity, they may cause liver dysfunction, particularly if alcohol is consumed—even in moderation.

Option 2:

If simple analgesics are not effective, we recommend combination analgesics, such as Anacin and Excedrin (Table 9–2). The caffeine in these products helps constrict blood vessels, enhances the pain relieving effect, and helps to improve absorption of medication through the stomach lining.

(Note that some other off-the-shelf preparations use "sinus" in their names and contain ingredients that constrict blood vessels. These may be useful in mild to moderate migraine or a mild sinus-type headache.)

Option 3:

If combination medications are not effective, we prescribe more potent medications such as nonsteroidal anti-inflammatory drugs or one that contains isometheptene, which constricts blood vessels; acetaminophen to relieve pain; and dichloralphenazone, which is a mild tranquilizer (Midrin).

Table 9–2: Off-the-Shelf Combination Analgesics

		Ingredients		
(mg)	Aspirin (mg)	Acetamino-phen (mg)	Caffeine (mg)	Other
Anacin	400		32	
Anacin (max. strength)	500		32	
BC-Powders	650		32	Salicylamide 195
Bufferin	324			Aluminum glycinate and magnesium carbonate
Cope	421		32	Magnesium hydroxide 50 and aluminum hydroxide 50
Excedrin (extra-strength)	250	250	65	
Excedrin PM		500		Diphenhydramine citrate 38
Midol Caplet	454		32.4	Cinnamedrine HCl 14.9
Percogesic		325		Phenyltoloxamine citrate 30
Vanquish	227	194	33	Aluminum hydroxide 50 and magnesium hydroxide 50

Prescription NSAIDs, which should be taken with food, can be helpful in treating a tension-type headache or mild migraine. For a listing of NSAIDs, refer to Table 9–3. Prescription NSAIDs may work better than those available off the shelf. At The New England Center for Headache we usually prescribe the following: naproxen sodium (Anaprox); ketoprofen (Orudis); meclofenamate (Meclomen); and flurbiprofen (Ansaid).

NSAID dose. The standard dose for prescription NSAIDs is 2 tablets or capsules initially followed by 2 more in 1 hour if necessary, with a maximum of 4 per day, 3 days per week.

Side effects. Patients may experience stomach pain, heartburn, and gastrointestinal bleeding (look for dark or tarry stools).

Table 9–3: Combination Analgesics Containing Butalbital

Drug/Components	Size (mg)	Recommended Dosage
Fiorinal		1–2 tablets q4h as needed;
Butalbital	50	no more than 6/day
Aspirin	325	
Caffeine	40	
Fioricet/Esgic		1–2 tablets q4h as needed;
Butalbital	50	no more than 6/day
Acetaminophen	325	
Caffeine	40	
Phrenilin		1–2 tablets q4h as needed;
Butalbital	50	no more than 6/day
Acetaminophen	325	

Midrin may be effective early in a mild migraine attack and has so few side effects that we use it in older children.

Dose. The dose of Midrin is 1 or 2 capsules at the start of a headache, followed by 1 or 2 more in 1 hour if the headache persists. Patients should take no more than 5 capsules in a day; use of Midrin should be limited to 3 days per week.

Side effects. Side effects of Midrin include occasional dizziness, drowsiness, or gastrointestinal symptoms.

Warning: Dangerous drug interactions could occur if Midrin is taken with a monoamine oxidase (MAO) inhibitor antidepressant (see page 46) such as phenelzine (Nardil) or tranylcypromine (Parnate).

Option 4:

If the above three options do not provide adequate relief, we prescribe medications that contain the short-acting barbiturate, butalbital. Refer to Table 9–3 for the names, ingredients, and recommended doses of butalbital-containing medications. If used frequently, any of these can cause dependence and rebound headache. Those that contain acetaminophen instead of aspirin are easier on the stomach; combinations that contain codeine are more potent pain relievers, but they are more likely to produce dependency.

Table 9–4: Antidepressants

Generic (Brand) Names		Generic (Brand) Names	
Tricyclics and Tetracyclics		*Selective Serotonin Reuptake Inhibitors* (SSRIs)	
Amitriptyline	(Elavil)	Fluoxetine	(Prozac)
Doxepin	(Sinequan, Adapin)	Sertraline	(Zoloft)
Nortriptyline	(Pamelor, Aventyl)	Paroxetine	(Paxil)
Desipramine	(Norpramin)		
Trazodone	(Desyrel)	*Miscellaneous*	
Imipramine	(Tofranil)	Bupropion	(Wellbutrin)
Amoxapine	(Asendin)	Venlafaxine	(Effexor)
Protriptyline	(Vivactil)	Nefazodone	(Serzone)
Maprotiline	(Ludiomil)		
Clomipramine	(Anafranil)	*MAOIs*	
		Phenelzine	(Nardil)
		Isocarboxazid	(Marplan)
		Tranylcypromine	(Parnate)

Dose. One or 2 tablets of butalbital-containing medications taken initially, and 1 or 2 again, in 2 to 4 hours, if necessary. Exceeding the daily limits listed in Table 9–3 may cause rebound headache or dependency.

Side effects. Butalbital-containing medications may cause drowsiness, poor coordination, and slurred speech.

Warning: Do not drink alcohol, drive, or operate machinery after taking these medications.

Option 5:

We prescribe opiates for our patients as back-up medication when necessary. Some rapid- to medium-acting opiates are oxycodone (Oxy IR), hydromorphone (Dilaudid), and butorphanol tartrate (Stadol nasal spray). Long-acting opiates are fentanyl (Duragesic patch), oxycodone (Oxycontin), and morphine sulfate (Kadian or MS Contin). When appropriate, we prescribe butorphanol tartrate nasal spray (Stadol NS) because it is easy for patients to use and permits home treatment of severe pain.

Side effects.   Drowsiness is a well-known opiate side effect, so plan to stay in after taking a dose. Since opiates may help you sleep, they are particularly useful for night-time headaches. Other side effects include nausea, vomiting, and dizziness.

Warning: Butorphanol may inactivate other opiates. Use this medication with caution if you are taking other medications that cause drowsiness. Overuse of any opiate can cause dependency. Use of opiates should be carefully controlled and limited to two days a week.

Option 6:

Other medications for tension-type headache include *muscle relaxants* such as carisoprodol (Soma), methocarbamol (Robaxin), cyclobenzaprine hydrochloride (Flexeril), metaxalone (Skelaxin), diazepam (Valium), and clonazepam (Klonopin), which is also used as an anticonvulsant, and which may be beneficial for patients whose headaches are associated with neck pain and muscle spasm. Baclofen (Lioresal) and tizanidine (Zanaflex) are highly potent anti-spasticity drugs typically used in patients with cerebral palsy and multiple sclerosis. They may be helpful in some patients with tension-type headaches and muscle spasm.

Dexamethasone (Decadron or Dexasone*),* which is a *steroid*, can be used if all else fails. It should be used only once or twice per month because frequent use of steroids can produce serious side effects.

Dose.   We prescribe a single 4-mg tablet, which may be repeated in 3 hours if the first dose is not effective.

Side effects.   Occasional use may cause reddening of the face and a slight increase in blood pressure. Excessive use produces multiple side effects, including loss of bone strength, ulcers, and joint deterioration.

Warning: Patients with uncontrolled high blood pressure and those with active ulcer disease should avoid use of steroids.

A tension-type headache that becomes severe may cause mild nausea. Our preferred antinausea medications are promethazine (Phenergan), taken by mouth or as a suppository, or oral metoclopramide (Reglan). Phenergan is more likely than Reglan to make you drowsy and help you sleep; Reglan keeps you alert, but can cause mild agitation.

Preventive Treatment of Chronic Tension-Type Headache

If you suffer from chronic tension-type headache and have headache most days of the week, a daily preventive medication may help. Antidepressant drugs, which increase serotonin levels, are the best way to treat chronic tension-type headache. Drugs from each of the three major categories: the *tricyclic and tetracyclic antidepressants* (TCAs), the *selective serotonin reuptake inhibitors* (SSRIs), and the *monoamine oxidase (MAO) inhibitors* may be effective for these headaches.

Antidepressants (see Table 9–4) should be chosen both for their ability to increase serotonin levels and for other effects, such as drowsiness, which may be helpful for some patients.

Tricyclic Antidepressants

Amitriptyline (Elavil) has been the gold standard for treatment of chronic headache, but its use may be limited by some of its side effects. At our Center, we prescribe antidepressants for patients with chronic tension-type headache as follows: for patients who have trouble sleeping through the night, awaken early in the morning, and who may be depressed— doxepin (Sinequan), amitriptyline (Elavil), or trazodone (Desyrel), which is neither a TCA nor an SSRI. Less sedating tricyclic agents include nortriptyline (Pamelor), desipramine (Norpramin), imipramine (Tofranil), and protriptyline (Vivactil). Imipramine and protriptyline have the least sedating effects and can be given in the morning. Two to 4 weeks of treatment may be required before patients notice an improvement in their headaches.

Dose. Sinequan is started at 10 mg, 1 to 2 hours before bedtime and is raised 10 mg every sixth night, until a total of 50 mg or 5 capsules is reached. This is an average dose and may have to be adjusted up or down. All medications are started at low doses and raised gradually to avoid side effects.

Side effects. All these medications have possible side effects, the most distressing of which are increased appetite, weight gain, drowsiness in the morning, dry mouth, and constipation. Blurred vision, sexual dysfunction, and urinary hesitancy occur less frequently.

Warning: Do not use these TCAs if you have heart rhythm irregularities, glaucoma, or experience difficulty urinating.

Selective Serotonin Reuptake Inhibitors (SSRIs)

The three most frequently prescribed SSRIs are fluoxetine (Prozac), sertraline (Zoloft), and paroxetine (Paxil) (see Table 9–4). SSRIs tend to have fewer side effects than the TCAs and are less likely to cause drowsiness and weight gain.

Dose. A patient taking fluoxetine would start with 10 mg each morning for 2 weeks, after which the dose could be raised to 20 mg if no side effects occur. Maximum benefit occurs between 3 to 6 weeks, and few people experience significant side effects. Higher doses may be necessary. Fluoxetine is long acting and remains in the body for days after administration has been discontinued.

Side effects. Mild agitation or hyperactivity shortly following the morning dose is the most common side effect associated with the SSRIs; this usually disappears within 2 weeks. Insomnia, tremor, difficulty having an orgasm, or other sexual dysfunction may occur. On rare occasions, SSRIs can make patients feel "off" psychologically. These drugs may cause depression or an increase in headache. Patients who notice drowsiness should take SSRIs at night. Weight loss is more common than weight gain, though either may occur.

Warning: SSRIs should be used cautiously in severely depressed patients and must not be used with MAO inhibitors.

Monoamine Oxidase Inhibitors (MAOIs)

When none of the above agents are helpful in preventing tension-type headache, a monoamine oxidase inhibitor (MAOI) such as phenelzine (Nardil) can be tried (see Table 9–4). Patients who take MAOIs must eliminate foods that contain tyramine from their diets to avoid drastic changes in blood pressure. The dietary restrictions are easy to follow.

Dose. Nardil is started with early morning doses of 15 mg, eventually building over the course of 1 month to a maximum dose of 30 mg in the morning and 30 mg at lunch time.

Side effects. Insomnia, weight gain, and changes in blood pressure are the major side effects.

Warnings: MAOIs should not be taken with Midrin, Demerol, and some other opiates, off-the-shelf cold medicines, and foods that contain tyramine (cheese, red wine, liver, etc.). When taking an MAOI, tricyclic antidepressants should be used with great caution, if at all, and SSRIs and the triptans (e.g., sumatriptan) are not to be used.

If none of the above antidepressant medications are helpful in treating chronic tension-type headache, other preventive medications may be tried (see page 48).

TREATMENT OF MIGRAINE ATTACKS

Option 1:

At any step, a triptan may completely and rapidly relieve pain and associated symptoms, and should be considered for migraine attacks of any intensity (see page 58). If caught early in its course, an acute migraine attack can be treated in much the same way as an acute tension-type headache (see page 37) with single-agent analgesics such as aspirin, acetaminophen (Tylenol), ibuprofen (Advil), ketoprofen (Orudis KT), or naproxen sodium (Aleve).

Option 2:

If the medications listed above are not effective, combination medications that contain aspirin, acetaminophen, and caffeine (Excedrin, Anacin) can be tried. If a caffeine-containing combination product is not available, try drinking a cup of coffee (which contains about 100 mg of caffeine) to constrict blood vessels and enhance the pain-relieving effect of aspirin.

Option 3:

Treatment is the same as in acute tension-type headache (see page 37). Nonsteroidal anti-inflammatory drugs (NSAIDs) may be helpful.

Option 4:

The next stronger category of medication to try is the butalbital-containing medicines which are more frequently used for tension-type headache (see Table 9–3). The best way to stop an acute migraine attack is to treat the underlying migraine process with *specific migraine medication.*

The Triptans

The introduction of *sumatriptan* (Imitrex in North America/ Imigran in Europe) in the early 1990s represented this century's most significant advance in migraine therapy. Sumatriptan rapidly terminates a migraine attack while eliminating associated symptoms such as nausea, vomiting, and light and sound sensitivity. It is associated with minimal side effects, has brought relief to millions of migraine sufferers worldwide, and has greatly enhanced quality of life due to its effectiveness and rapid restoration of ability to function. Sumatriptan has, in effect, become the standard against which newer antimigraine drugs will be measured.

As a result of sumatriptan's resounding success, several other pharmaceutical companies are developing similar compounds in the hope of offering faster relief more consistently, fewer side effects, and a lower rate of headache recurrence (headache returning within 24 hours).

As a class, the triptans constrict blood vessels in the head and reverse inflammation around those vessels in the meninges (brain covering). They may, however, constrict other blood vessels and thus should not be given to patients with coronary artery disease, stroke, uncontrolled high blood pressure, and two rare forms of migraine known as hemiplegic migraine (stroke-like symptoms) and basilar artery migraine (associated with poor coordination and fainting).

For those with risk factors for coronary disease (men over 40, women past menopause, obese patients, patients with high cholesterol, diabetics, smokers, family history of coronary disease in a close relative at an early age, and nonexercisers), it is advisable to administer these agents for the first time in a doctor's office. Blood pressure should be measured and a cardiogram should be done prior to, and following administration, in addition to monitoring for side effects following dosage. Any patient reporting chest pain or pressure should be carefully evaluated before continuing to use these drugs. Properly prescribed for appropriate patients with migraine, the triptans are safe and effective.

Side effects of the triptans are generally mild and short-lived and include tingling sensations in fingers, warmth, flushing, chest and/or neck pressure, and rarely chest pain. Patients who experience lightheadedness and fatigue should rest for a short time after dosing.

Though these medications may eliminate the attack, headache may return within 24 hours with sufficient severity to require a repeat dose. In reporting the usefulness of these medications to your doctor, you should include the following information:

1. How long does it take before you feel the drug beginning to work?
2. How long before you feel significant relief and can return to your usual activities?
3. How much better is the pain (for example: 70% or 100% improvement)?
4. What percentage of the time does the drug work? (8 out of 10 times equals 80%)
5. In what percentage of attacks does the headache return within 24 hours (% recurrence)?
6. If the headache recurs, how long does it take to return (time to recurrence)?

Like all medications prescribed by your doctor, the triptans should be taken only as directed. Maintaining good control of migraine can help reduce the need for emergency department and physician visits, and may improve overall quality of life.

A brief review of information available for each of these medicines follows (see page 51). Since a wider variety of effective medications will be available in a variety of delivery systems (tablets, injections, nasal sprays, and preparations that dissolve instantly on your tongue without the need for water), do not lose hope if you do not respond to one preparation or have uncomfortable side effects; you may do well with another—or even the same one—for your next attack.

Sumatriptan (Imitrex/Imigran) is available in three dosage forms: injection, tablet, and nasal spray. Each injection delivers 6 mg via a novel autoinjector; this is the most rapidly acting form. Injection can be repeated once if the headache returns with sufficient severity. Maximum dose is two injections in 24 hours. Seventy percent of the time patients feel relief within 1 hour and 80% of the time within 2 hours. The average percentage recurrence in worldwide studies is about 40%, with average time to recurrence of 14 hours.

In a study conducted by our group at The New England Center for Headache in Stamford, Connecticut, and published in the journal *Headache*, we reported an 84% success rate in the first 100 patients who tried Imitrex injection. Eighty-one percent of the patients said it worked better than anything they had previously tried for migraine, and many termed it "a miracle drug." Forty-six percent of our patients had a recurrent headache between 8 and 15 hours after the first dose; this was treated effectively with a second dose. No patient stopped the drug due to side effects.

Sumatriptan is available in the United States also as 25- and 50-mg tablets. The 50-mg dose is often more effective than the 25-mg, and a few patients require 75 or 100 mg as a starting dose; maximum dosage is 300 mg in 24 hours. The average response rate at 2 hours is about 55% and 70% at 4 hours. We recommend taking another dose if there is no response 2 to 3 hours after the first dose. Patients whose starting dose was 25 mg and who require a repeat dose to get rid of the headache should start with 50 mg for the next and subsequent attacks.

Sumatriptan nasal spray is available in 5 mg and 20 mg single-dose units; dosage is a single spray in one nostril. Most patients will respond to the 20-mg dose, which works faster than a tablet. Taste disturbance is the most common side effect, followed by nausea, vomiting, fatigue, and flushing.

Zolmitriptan (Zomig) is currently available in the United Kingdom and Sweden, and should be available in the United States in the near future. Clinical studies show a 46% response within 1 hour, 65% at 2 hours, and 78% at 4 hours. Forty-five percent of patients are totally pain free at 4 hours after dosage. The 2.5-mg dose can be doubled if required. Representative of the newer triptans, zolmitriptan may offer patients a more consistently reliable medication that is effective in a broad range of migraine and patient types. It works well in menstrual migraine and in migraine present on awakening. As with all triptans, zolmitriptan must be used cautiously in patients with cardiovascular risk factors. The most common side effects are nausea, dizziness, sleepiness, and tingling in the fingers; these effects are mild and transient. Recurrence rate is just under 30%. A nasal spray is being developed.

Naratriptan, known as Naramig in Europe and Amerge in the US, should become available in the United States as a 2.5-mg tablet in the near future. Its developers expect it to be better tolerated, with a lower rate of recurrent headache and side effects than its older sibling, sumatriptan (Imitrex).

Other agents likely to be available over the next few years include rizatriptan (Maxalt) which may have an early onset of action and high rate of efficacy, eletriptan which may work in a higher percentage of patients, VML 251 which appears to have a low recurrence rate, and almotriptan.

Ergots

Ergotamine tartrate (Cafergot, Wigraine) has been in use for over 50 years as a specific migraine agent. Rectal suppositories are better absorbed and more effective than tablets in the treatment of headache. In Europe, this method is the preferred route of administration.

Dose. We recommend two ergotamine (Wigraine) tablets at the start of a migraine attack, followed by two more tablets in an hour if needed. If the suppository form is used, start with 1/4 (Cafergot) and repeat in an hour if needed. Refer to antinauseants for recommendations about pretreatment to prevent nausea. We instruct patients to use ergotamine only 1 day per week, 2 days maximum. The only exception is that women may use it for 3 consecutive days during menstrual periods.

Side effects. Side effects include nausea and vomiting, and some patients experience tingling in the fingers and toes, chest pain, and muscle cramps.

Dihydroergotamine (D.H.E. 45), which is chemically related to ergotamine tartrate, is also effective and is less likely to cause nausea. Originally available only as an injectable solution, the new nasal spray form, Migranal, is available in Canada. It should soon be available in the United States.

Dose. The initial injectable dose is 1 mg, which may be repeated in 2 hours if needed. The headache is not likely to recur once it disappears. For the nasal spray, we recommend one spray in each nostril as an initial dose, repeated in 10 minutes. These four sprays contain 0.5 mg each for a total dose of 2 mg; this dosage may be repeated after 1 hour. DHE is less likely to cause recurrent or rebound headache than the triptans, and can be used several days per week.

Side effects. The most frequent side effects from the nasal spray seem to be occasional stuffiness of the nose or muscle cramps.

Warnings: Patients who take macrolide antibiotics (erythromycin and azithromycin—Zithromax) or have coronary artery disease, hypertension, or peripheral vascular disease, or who could be pregnant, should not take DHE.

If none of the above are helpful, opiates (narcotics) may be required. With the exception of butorphanol nasal spray (Stadol NS), which is effective in relieving headache pain, we prefer not to use stronger opiates (narcotics), (see page 43). We recommend that butorphanol be used for rescue if other specific agents have not been effective or cannot be used. Dosing recommendations must be followed carefully.

Other medications used for migraine are the *antiemetics*. Antiemetics combat nausea due to migraine or which occurs as a side effect of specific medication such as ergotamine tartrate (Cafergot). If you need to stay alert and go back to work, we recommend taking metoclopramide (Reglan), about 15 minutes before an ergotamine-type specific medication. If you need to sleep or can remain at home, promethazine (Phenergan) can be taken by mouth or as a suppository. Other antiemetics that may help include prochlorperazine (Compazine), trimethobenzamide (Tigan), chlorpromazine (Thorazine), hydroxyzine (Vistaril), and an off-the-shelf liquid preparation, Emetrol. Emetrol can be added to any of the previously mentioned antiemetics, and can be repeated every 15 to 30 minutes. The newer ondansetron (Zofran) is extremely effective.

Migraine patients with anxiety may feel better on *benzodiazepine minor tranquilizers* such as lorazepam (Ativan), alprazolam (Xanax), diazepam (Valium), and clorazepate (Tranxene). Although these drugs may relieve anxiety and promote relaxation, they may be addictive and may worsen headache syndromes. Buspirone (Buspar) is not addictive and can be used daily for treatment of anxiety.

Lidocaine in the form of nasal drops can sometimes rapidly stop a one-sided migraine attack. It is currently being evaluated for this use.

PREVENTIVE (PROPHYLACTIC) TREATMENT OF MIGRAINE

When three or more severe migraine attacks occur per month, if each attack lasts for 2 days or more, or if attacks are difficult to treat with the symptomatic and specific acute-care migraine medications already mentioned, then daily preventive medications should be given to block migraine attacks. There are several categories that can be used; some patients will do better with one type of medication over another.

Beta-Blockers

Beta-blockers may work by preventing dilation or swelling of arteries. Of the many beta-blockers, propranolol (Inderal), atenolol (Tenormin), metoprolol (Lopressor, Toprol-XL), nadolol (Corgard), and timolol (Blocadren) are the most effective for prevention of migraine. Those we most frequently prescribe are atenolol, nadolol, and propranolol.

Dose. Our patients take propranolol 10 to 20 mg twice a day, increasing by 10 to 20 mg every 5 days up to a dose of about 60 to 80 mg. Some patients take more than 360 mg daily. If a patient does well on short-acting propranolol in divided doses, we may then switch to the longer-acting form.

Side effects. Potential side effects include fatigue, depression, impotence, reduced blood pressure and pulse rate, weight gain, reduced tolerance to physical activity, and dizziness on standing.

Warnings: These drugs should not be given to people with asthma, diabetes, low blood sugar (hypoglycemia), slow heart rate, low blood pressure, and severe depression. They should also not be used in severe cases of migraine accompanied by weakness on one side of the body or other evidence of focal brain dysfunction. Patients who need to stop taking beta-blockers should taper the dosage gradually over several days to prevent rapid heartbeat.

Calcium Channel Blockers

Calcium channel blockers prevent calcium from entering certain cells in the brain and muscles. This, in turn, prevents blood vessels from constricting, which blocks part of the migraine process. The most widely used calcium blocker for migraine in the United States is verapamil (Calan, Isoptin), followed by diltiazem (Cardizem). Others such as nisoldipine (Sular), nicardipine (Cardene), and flunarizine (Sibelium, available only in Canada and Europe) may also be used.

Dose. Verapamil is usually started at 40 mg per day and increased quickly to 40 mg three times per day. After that, dosage can be gradually increased to 80–160 mg three times per day.

Side effects. Constipation and fluid retention are the most common side effects; heart effects, low blood pressure, drowsiness, and dizziness may also occur.

Warnings. Patients with significant cardiac problems should not use calcium channel blockers; those who take other blood pressure medications—especially beta-blockers—should use them with caution.

Antidepressants

See page 44 for a discussion of antidepressants, which are often helpful in reducing tension-type headache and can be used in patients who have migraine associated with tension-type headache or depression.

Anticonvulsants

Anticonvulsants, which are used in seizure disorders such as epilepsy, may be useful for prevention of migraine. Divalproex sodium (Depakote in the United States, Epival in Canada) effectively reduces the frequency of migraine in many patients, even if they have not responded to other medications. Other anticonvulsants such as phenytoin (Dilantin) and carbamazepine (Tegretol) have not been as effective, although children may respond to phenytoin better than adults. Gabapentin (Neurontin) may be an effective migraine preventive agent and is being tested in the United States. Lamotrigine (Lamictal) is also undergoing testing.

Dose. If started at low doses, and increased slowly over time, divalproex sodium (Depakote) is much less likely to cause side effects. It is safer for use in adults than in young children. We have adult patients start with 125 mg of divalproex sodium once per day and slowly increase the dose until they reach 750 to 1000 mg per day in two divided doses. Blood levels of the drug should be checked to assess when therapeutic levels have been reached, and occasional blood tests are important to make certain that liver function and blood count remain normal.

Side effects.   Side effects may include weight gain, hair loss, tremor, and sedation. Reducing the dosage or stopping the drug for a short period, then restarting it at lower doses, usually reverses side effects.

Warning: Women who are pregnant, or who may become pregnant, should not take divalproex sodium because it can cause serious spinal cord defects in the fetus. It should not be used in anyone with liver disease and should be given cautiously to children. It should be used cautiously in combination with barbiturates such as phenobarbital and butalbital-containing medications.

Note that phenytoin, carbamazepine, and some other anticonvulsants may reduce the effectiveness of oral contraceptives (birth control pills), particularly the newer ones with very low estrogen content.

Serotonin$_2$ Antagonists (Blockers)

Cyproheptadine (Periactin) is an antihistamine that blocks serotonin$_2$ receptors. It is effective in preventing migraine attacks in children, but somewhat less so in adults.

Dose.   Cyproheptadine is available in tablets and liquid form. The starting dose is 1/4 of a 4-mg tablet (1 mg), 1 to 2 hours before bedtime; dosage can be slowly increased to a total of 2 to 4 tablets.

Side effects.   Children tolerate cyproheptadine well and experience few side effects. Adults, however, may become drowsy or have increased appetite with weight gain. Drowsiness may be beneficial for patients who sleep poorly.

Warnings: Patients who take monoamine oxidase inhibitors (MAOIs; see page 46) or who have glaucoma, enlarged prostate, or obstruction of the bladder should not take cyproheptadine.

Methysergide (Sansert) is one of the oldest preventive migraine medications and works both by blocking serotonin$_2$ receptors and by constricting blood vessels.

Dose. Available as a 2-mg tablet, methysergide is usually taken 3 times a day.

Side effects. At the higher doses, side effects may be nausea, muscle cramps, and abdominal pain. Patients who use methysergide should stop taking it for 1 month after 6 months' use to avoid its most serious side effect, retroperitoneal fibrosis (scarring—an overgrowth of the filmy connective tissue around certain organs deep in the abdomen.) This usually disappears when methysergide is discontinued.

Warnings: Patients with heart problems such as coronary artery disease or peripheral vascular disease, history of inflammation in the leg veins, or stomach ulcers should not take methysergide.

Methylergonovine (Methergine) is a related ergot that can be taken daily for prevention of migraine. It blocks serotonin$_2$ receptors and constricts blood vessels, as does methysergide.

Dose. The starting dose is a 0.2-mg tablet once per day, which is slowly raised to three times per day. The maximum dose is usually 2 tablets three times per day.

Side effects. Possible side effects include muscle aches (cramps in women), hallucinations (rarely), and signs of constricted blood vessels (such as chest pain).

Warnings: Methylergonovine should not be used by anyone with heart disease, arterial disease, vein disease, high blood pressure, or possibility of pregnancy; it should not be taken continuously for more than 6 months without a drug holiday.

Alpha$_2$-Adrenoceptor Agonists (Stimulators)

Clonidine (Catapres) may help prevent migraine. It works best in women who are perimenopausal and in patients who are being withdrawn from opiates (narcotics) and nicotine. It blocks the release of a chemical called norepinephrine from the brain stem.

Dose. The usual dose of clonidine is half of a 0.1-mg tablet, once or twice per day; the maximum dose is 3 tablets per day. Available also as a skin patch (Catapres-TTS # 1, 2, and 3), the starting dose is a 0.1-mg patch worn for 1 week at a time.

Side effects. Side effects include drowsiness, dizziness, and decreased blood pressure.

Warnings: Patients on blood pressure medications, and those who feel drowsy and dizzy should not take clonidine.

Lithium

Lithium carbonate, which is usually used for cluster headache, can sometimes be helpful in migraine—especially a rare form known as cyclical migraine. It works on cell membranes deep in the brain. Those who take lithium should drink plenty of fluids to avoid dehydration and should limit salt (sodium) intake. Blood levels should be monitored periodically.

Dose. The starting dose is 300 mg once per day and can be raised to two or three times per day.

Warnings: Lithium carbonate should be used cautiously in combination with calcium channel blockers and should not be taken with diuretics.

Stimulant Medications

Since it is difficult to determine which patients will respond to stimulant medication such as dextroamphetamine (Dexedrine), methylphenidate (Ritalin), or pemoline (Cylert), they are usually reserved for patients who have not responded to other medications.

NSAIDs

The nonsteroidal anti-inflammatory medications can be taken with food to help decrease the frequency of migraine. They may be highly effective, even when other drugs have not worked (see Table 9–3). Patients should watch for stomach pain. These medications may work well for women whose headaches increase during the menstrual periods or ovulation because the drugs inhibit the production of prostaglandins, which cause inflammation and pain.

Hormonal Treatment

Hormonal regulation and other techniques have been tried in women whose headaches occur mostly around their menstrual periods or when they ovulate. For a further discussion of headache and the menstrual cycle, refer to Chapter 14.

Sometimes the diuretic acetazolamide (Diamox) can decrease the production of spinal fluid and improve headache. The starting dose is 125 mg three times per day; the side effects are tingling around the mouth and at the tips of the fingers as well as increased urination. A variety of *vitamin and herbal preparations* that may be used are described in Chapter 10.

ACUTE TREATMENT OF CLUSTER HEADACHE

A cluster headache attack is best treated by breathing pure oxygen for up to 20 minutes through a loosely fitting mask that covers the mouth and nose. We recommend that patients sit on comfortable furniture, leaning forward. Ergotamine tartrate can be given by mouth (Wigraine), under the tongue, or as rectal suppository (Cafergot) to stop an attack. An injection of dihydroergotamine (D.H.E. 45) is very helpful, and nasal spray preparations (Imitrex and Migranal) may be helpful, too. A self-administered injection of sumatriptan (Imitrex) can rapidly stop a cluster headache and has been approved by the Food and Drug Administration (FDA). Daily use of opiates is not recommended, due to risk of dependency and rebound headache. Spraying cocaine into the nose may be effective, but the drug is highly addictive and should rarely be used. Lidocaine (in spite of the "caine" in its name, lidocaine is not addictive) nasal drops may be helpful, and capsaicin (extract of red peppers) can be effective but may work better when used daily as a preventive treatment.

PREVENTIVE TREATMENT OF CLUSTER HEADACHES

Verapamil, a calcium channel blocker, appears at present to be the most effective preventive treatment for cluster headache. The dose is an 80-mg tablet three times per day; 4 to 6 such tablets per day are occasionally required.

Prednisone, a steroid, starting at 60 mg per day, tapering gradually to nothing over a period of 2 to 3 weeks, may prevent attacks. If, however, the cluster period has not ended when the steroid dose has decreased to a critically low level, the cluster headaches will return.

Warning: Long-term use of prednisone (or any steroid) may cause numerous side effects and should be avoided.

Ergotamine tartrate (Wigraine), 1 tablet once or twice per day for several weeks may prevent attacks from occurring. Keep in mind that this treatment is not used in migraine, as it increases the frequency of migraine attacks by causing a rebound syndrome.

Lithium carbonate may also prevent cluster headache; 300 mg twice daily usually brings relief. Refer to precautions under migraine prevention.

Methysergide (Sansert), 2 mg three times per day and methylergonovine (Methergine), 0.2 mg three times per day, can be taken daily to prevent cluster headache for up to 6 months.

Divalproex sodium (Depakote) may prevent cluster headache for some patients. We start with 125 mg per day, and increase the dose to 750 mg in two divided doses.

When no other medications have worked, Indomethacin (Indocin), an NSAID, is surprisingly helpful in some patients with cluster headache. Patients start at 25 mg three times per day with meals; it must be used with caution to reduce risk of ulcer. Some patients respond to acetazolamide (Diamox), starting at 125 mg three times per day.

Capsaicin, an extract of red peppers, has been investigated as a cluster headache preventive by David Marks, MD, of The New England Center for Headache. Results suggest that it can help reduce pain after about 5 days of daily application inside the nostril on the side of the pain. It is available without prescription as Zostrix HP (0.075%), but should be used only under a doctor's direction.

Patients with severe cluster headache who do not respond to outpatient therapy should be admitted to an inpatient headache unit for more aggressive care, which usually includes intravenous D.H.E. 45.

CONCLUSION

Many medications are available for acute and preventive treatment of each type of headache. These, plus a variety of behavioral techniques, provide you and your doctor with the tools required to design a personalized program to help you conquer your headache.

At our Center, we share the belief of many clinicians that an appropriate combination of pharmacologic and nonpharmacologic (without medication) treatments can be more effective than either alone.

Nonpharmacologic treatment techniques can be classified as active and passive. Active techniques require patient involvement, responsibility, and participation, focusing on such activities as keeping headache calendars, making nutritional changes, exercising, practicing relaxation techniques, and modifying behavior that may contribute to headaches. With passive techniques, patients simply receive treatments without modifying their behavior.

ACTIVE TECHNIQUES

The underlying concept that patients' behavior is key to the continuation or relief of any illness is the basis of behavioral medicine. Doctors and patients should review issues that might stand in the way of successful treatment. Because we recognize how difficult it can be to make changes in lifestyles, we provide our patients with clear instructions and initiate discussions about potential pitfalls. This chapter reviews important active techniques that may help you to deal with your headaches.

Headache Calendar

Headache calendars are daily logs of anything that might relate to your headaches and are vital to appropriate treatment. As we discuss how to use a headache calendar, refer to Fig. 10–1a.

A headache calendar helps a patient record ongoing information about the frequency, intensity, and duration of headaches. It can also help patients monitor how and when to take medication, track its effectiveness, and document potential headache triggers. It also helps to show any relationship between headaches and a woman's menstrual cycle. Each calendar represents 1 month of headache activity. We ask our patients to record headache intensity, timing, medications used and triggers.

Both preventive and abortive medications must be listed. When listing abortive medications, patients record the degree of relief obtained from 0=no relief to 3=complete relief. Under the heading "nonmedication," patients record exercise, relaxation activities, and other recommended techniques. Figure 10–1b shows the reverse side of our calendar, which lists potential headache triggers. Patients record these under "triggers." To record the days of menstrual flow, women also enter Xs in the boxes labeled "period." Finally, all medications—both prescription (from us and from other physicians) and off-the-shelf medications—must be recorded.

These calendars also help doctors to monitor their patients' progress. The first calendar is used as a baseline, and, at follow-up visits, we review any changes in the calendar, and record them as percent change from the baseline. Patients who take frequent doses or large quantities of pain relievers or ergotamine, use the calendars to follow a specific program, the goal of which is to decrease and eliminate daily use of these medications.

Relaxation Techniques

The goal of relaxation techniques is to reduce the "fight/flight" response and levels of substances the body produces in response to stress. Also used in biofeedback therapy, deep, rhythmic breathing techniques are the basis of all relaxation strategies. To try deep, rhythmic breathing, sit in a comfortable chair in a quiet environment; loosen your collar and belt, and close your eyes. Inhale (breathe in) deeply and slowly, making sure that your abdomen moves more than your chest. At first, inhale to a count of three, working your way up to ten as you master the technique. When you reach your peak,

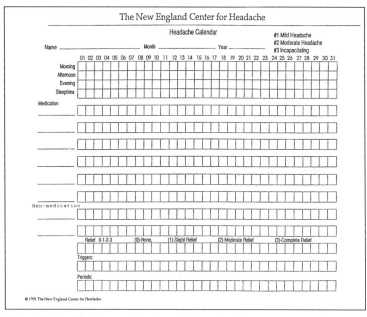

Figure 10–1a: The front of the headache calendar used at our Center.

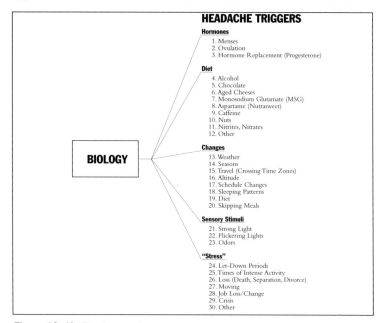

Figure 10–1b: The back of the calendar.

hold it for a second or so and then exhale (let it out) slowly to the same count. Alan Turin, PhD, of Boston suggests that patients focus on inhaling in "relaxation" and exhaling out, "tension" as they do the exercise.

Progressive relaxation.   Tense your toes slowly as you inhale to a slow count and then relax them as you exhale. Then move up your body, alternately tensing and relaxing muscles of your calves, thighs, buttocks, abdomen, back, fingers, arms, shoulders, neck, and—finally—the muscles of your head and jaws.

Autogenic training.   Try repeating a series of phrases to yourself to suggest changes such as feeling warmth and heaviness. You might, for example, repeat, "my legs are warm and heavy," while associating this with a pleasant feeling. Move up the body as described for progressive relaxation.

Visual imagery.   Help to relax the head and neck muscles by visualizing them as tight, scrunched, uneven, crooked, crossing lines. Then focus on making the lines smoother, straighter, and evenly spaced. Visualize yourself on a sandy beach with your hands under the hot sand. Now feel the sand warm your hands.

Exercises that focus on warmth may help patients with migraine, many of whom tend to have cold hands and feet. Done successfully, visualization can divert blood flow from the head to the hands and/or feet while bringing on a state of relaxation.

Body scan.   Our colleagues at the New England Institute for Behavioral Medicine, Steven Baskin, PhD and Randall Weeks, PhD, teach their patients how to perform a "body scan." They suggest that their patients remain alert for signs of tension in the head, neck, shoulders, arms, or legs throughout the day. Without realizing it, many people hunch their shoulders, which creates muscle tension in the shoulders, neck, and head. Or they may contract muscles around the neck or head, or clench their jaws or fists. People who check for these signs of tension throughout the day may be able to reduce muscle tension and decrease the effects of stress on the body. This type of body scan can be accompanied by deep breathing and other relaxation techniques.

Get in the habit of stopping what you are doing once every hour to check for signs of muscle tension and to take a quick deep-breathing/relaxation break. Relax with gentle neck rolls; allow your chin to fall to your chest, then gently rotate your head right and left 5 or 10 times. If you work at a computer for hours at a time, take a few minutes every hour or so to cup your hands over your eyes, giving your eyes a chance to rest.

Biofeedback. Biofeedback is commonly used in the treatment of both tension-type headache and migraine. It has not been found useful in cluster headache. Biofeedback may be administered by a clinical psychologist trained in the technique, or by a trained biofeedback technician. Effective in children and adults, the goal is to reduce symptoms and ultimately to eliminate the need for feedback.

Biofeedback is a "return of information" about biologic processes. It works because electronic equipment senses information such as temperature or muscle tension and gives you auditory or visual "feedback." Over time, the combination of feedback and reinforcement helps you to control muscle tension, temperature, and other functions.

Cognitive Therapy

Cognition means thinking. Many people have negative feelings, and they translate these into such statements as "I will never get rid of my headaches." Cognitive therapists believe that if you can change your thoughts, you can change the feelings associated with these thoughts. Cognitive therapy has proven successful in treating anxiety disorders and depression. It has also proven useful in treating headache disorders. Psychologists and other health-care professionals who practice cognitive therapy can help you challenge these negative thoughts, change your thinking, and ultimately change the way you feel. This can give you a more positive, optimistic, and ultimately a less destructive way to think, feel, and be.

Psychotherapy

Psychotherapy alone has not been found useful as a headache treatment. If, however, headaches are accompanied by psychological difficulties, marital problems, job-related difficulties, depression, anxiety, and other problems, psychotherapy can help.

Group therapy, particularly in the form of support groups, has been useful for headache sufferers as well as patients with a variety of chronic illnesses. Headache groups are currently being offered in cities throughout the United States by the American Council for Headache Education (ACHE) and the National Headache Foundation (NHF).

Lifestyle Changes

All of the techniques described in this chapter require you to review and modify various aspects of your lifestyle. Calendars can be useful in helping you to identify potential headache-provoking or stressful situations and trigger factors, including food. Remember to eat a healthful, balanced diet at regular times each day. Exercise is vital for reducing headache and maintaining good health. So is sleep.

Since many patients focus on others' needs but leave little time for themselves, we suggest that our patients use an appointment book to schedule time for themselves—"me time" and to keep the appointment.

PASSIVE TECHNIQUES

Acupuncture

Acupuncture, an ancient Asian healing art, involves placing needles in the skin at specific points. Acupuncture corrects what are termed imbalances between the two parts (yin and yang) of a life force known as Ch'i. Applied correctly, the needles cause minimal or no pain or discomfort. If you have no response after six or eight sessions, acupuncture probably will not work for you.

Acupressure

Acupressure is a technique based on acupuncture. Some have found using the thumb and forefinger to squeeze the web between the thumb and forefinger of the other hand effective in aborting migraine. For tension-type headache, pressure can be applied to the small indentations approximately midway between the outer border of the eye and the inner border of the ear and also at the back of the head.

Chiropractic Therapy

Chiropractic therapy is based on the theory that most diseases of the body are a result of misalignment of the vertebral column. The goal of the treatment is to realign the vertebrae through the use of manual techniques called "adjustments." Many neurologists question the validity of chiropractic therapy and are concerned that aggressive manipulation, or adjustments, of the neck may injure important structures such as the blood vessels that supply the brain.

Physical and Occupational Therapy

Physical therapy has been used in headache disorders and, in particular, in tension-type headache, where the neck and shoulder muscles may be involved. Heat and massage have been tried as muscle relaxants since antiquity, and newer techniques such as ultrasound, which deliver deep heat to muscles, have been shown to be helpful in reducing spasm and tenderness. Electrical stimulation may also be beneficial. Many patients may benefit from improvement in posture and gait, and these patients may be given appropriate exercises to do at home. Other treatments such as active and passive stretching increase the range of motion about the neck.

Some patients' occupations contribute to muscle tension. Computer users, administrative personnel, and telephone representatives may all develop tense muscles in their backs and necks as well as postural problems that contribute to tension-type headache. Frequent breaks and professional attention to posture may help.

Application of cold to the head may help to constrict dilated blood vessels, override pain transmission, numb the skin, and reduce metabolic activity in muscles, contributing to the relief of pain. Studies have shown, and many of our patients agree, that the headache ice-pillow is useful.

The molded pillow fits comfortably around the neck and back of the head and holds a frozen gel pack that ices the nape of the neck. Ice applied to the forehead, eyes, and temples can also be helpful, and some patients get relief by taking a warm shower.

Massage Therapy

Massage can reduce muscle tension in various parts of the body, and it can reduce headache. A variety of techniques are practiced by licensed massage therapists.

Trigger Point Injections

Occurring in various parts of the body, trigger points are small areas that feel like knots of muscle tissue; they are tender to touch and may refer pain to various areas of the head. The exact cause of trigger points is not fully understood. However, an injection of local anesthetic into these tender points can be helpful.

Transcutaneous Electrical Nerve Stimulation (TENS)

TENS blocks the transmission of the pain with electrodes placed on the skin *between pain and brain*. At this time, the results of TENS therapy for headache have been somewhat disappointing, though this therapy has proven more successful in treating other types of chronic pain. A new type of low-intensity stimulation to the ear lobe is being tested.

NATUROPATHY AND HOMEOPATHY

These two disciplines represent alternatives to traditional medical treatments and are attractive to some patients who want to avoid pharmacologic therapy. Naturopathy uses only natural substances in small amounts. Homeopathy uses natural substances as well as minute amounts of the active ingredients in some medications. Traditional physicians would view the amounts of these medications as far too small to produce a therapeutic response and term any effects a *placebo response*. All the same, many patients seem to have benefited from these approaches.

Herbal, Mineral, and Vitamin Therapies

Do **not** use any of the following without first checking with your doctor.

Feverfew.   A variety of herbal therapies has been used to prevent migraine, the most popular of which has been feverfew, which is derived from the chrysanthemum family of plants. A small, placebo-controlled trial, published in the *British Medical Journal* in 1985 suggests that it may, indeed, prevent migraine in some patients. Feverfew is available in several forms and dosages and is usually found in health food stores.

Magnesium.   Magnesium is a trace element found in the body. Some scientific evidence suggests that magnesium levels are lower in the brains of migraine patients. Use of magnesium to treat migraine is under study. We recommend using 400 mg per day if it does not produce diarrhea.

Vitamin therapies.   We suggest 50 mg of vitamin B6 and 400 international units of vitamin E daily. In April 1997, at an international meeting of neurologists in Boston, Professor Jean Schoenen of Belgium reported that vitamin B2 (riboflavin) proved significantly better than placebo in preventing headache when taken in a dose of 400 mg per day. High doses of vitamin A are not only potentially toxic, they may cause headache. Some say vitamin C helps headache; however, results are inconsistent.

Garlic and ginger.   Some patients have found that garlic and ginger have properties that might be useful in migraine.

Ginseng.   Ginseng is said to decrease tension and relieve headache. It is available as a tea and in capsules, tablets, and dried root powder. **Ginkgo Biloba** and **valerian root** have been touted as effective by patients.

Fish oil.   Although not a herbal remedy, fish oil is available without prescription. Some have found that regular doses appear to decrease the frequency of migraine. Fish oil may work by reducing platelet clumping, which some believe is an important factor in migraine.

CONCLUSION

A number of treatments alternative to pharmacological therapy are available. Some of these techniques may be helpful to you, and others may not. Keep in mind, however, that an immediate and permanent cure for migraine has not yet been discovered.

CHAPTER 11

DOCTOR-PATIENT RELATIONSHIP

We think an educated patient is a better patient. You should know as much as possible about your headaches, your treatment plan, and the medications you take. Sometimes the amount and type of information a patient receives are defined by the doctor–patient relationship.

Rotor and Hall in their book, *Doctors Talking with Patients/Patients Talking with Doctors,* describe a number of different types of doctor–patient relationships.

We feel that the mutualistic doctor–patient relationship yields the most positive treatment outcome. Thus, we urge you to find a physician who is open to this style and who will take the time to listen to you, hear your concerns, educate you, and give you feedback about your condition, treatment options, and medications.

Your doctor should accept the validity, reality, intensity, and quality of your pain. Does he/she:

1. accept your complaints, or dismiss them as unimportant?
2. take the time to listen to you?
3. understand headache? It is all right to ask if he or she sees many headache patients and what his/her success rate is. Does he or she have a board certification or affiliation with a medical school and/or work at a teaching hospital?
4. seem compassionate and understanding?
5. seem flexible about exploring a variety of treatment options?
6. take the time to discuss his or her findings, diagnosis, and treatment plan as well as alternative treatments?
7. answer your questions to your satisfaction?
8. tell you what to expect from treatment (prognosis)?
9. tell you what medication is being prescribed, how it works, how frequently to take it and when, and what

side effects it may cause? Your doctor should note significant drug interactions (including alcohol) and tell you what off-the-shelf medications to avoid. Did he or she say how long you will need to take the medication, how and when to reduce or increase dosage, and how or when to discontinue it?

10. describe to you any tests ordered and their purposes, and explain how the results will be used?

11. discuss with you nonpharmacologic interventions related to changes in your lifestyle? If so, has he or she expressed interest in how you plan to make these changes?

It is a good idea to write down all your questions before a visit to any doctor. These questions should include how to reach him or her during off-hours, or who covers when he or she is not on call. Be sure to ask whether your doctor has a specific "telephone time"—many do.

Remember, taking a cooperative, active role in the treatment of your headache improves your chances of success. Good doctor-patient communication is an important beginning.

EMERGENCY DEPARTMENT AND HOSPITAL TREATMENT

Your physician should give you several levels of headache treatment for home care to decrease the likelihood of your needing emergency care.

If you have to go to an emergency room, go with someone who can take you home; the staff might otherwise be reluctant to give you strong pain or antinausea medications. Although some emergency rooms are set up for headache patients, most put patients with headache in noisier, colder, brighter rooms than are ideal. You may also have a long wait. With this in mind, we suggest that you take with you a sweatshirt, dark glasses, and patience. Since emergency room staff may suspect headache patients of drug-seeking behavior, we provide our patients with cards that identify them as migraine sufferers and suggest appropriate treatment.

In a headache-friendly emergency room, you can expect to be ushered into a dim, quiet room, where you receive a blanket to keep you warm and a basin in case you vomit. The staff will evaluate you appropriately, and if you say you are having pain typical of one of your migraine attacks, you will probably be treated without further evaluation. If, however, you raise any of the red flags (see page 24) you may undergo further evaluation.

MIGRAINE TREATMENT

If you have intermittent migraine and need acute care, you are likely to receive either injectable dihydroergotamine (D.H.E. 45) or sumatriptan (Imitrex), which are the two best injectable medications currently available to abort a migraine.

Dihydroergotamine (D.H.E. 45)

DHE has been available for half a century and can be injected intramuscularly, intravenously, or under the skin

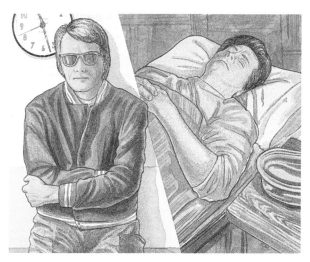

Figure 12–1: Headache patients in emergency rooms.

(subcutaneously). Given alone, DHE gets rid of headache for a long time and often reduces nausea. When our patients go to the Greenwich Hospital Emergency Department they usually receive three injections: D.H.E. 45, Decadron (a steroid), and promethazine (Phenergan) for nausea.

Sumatriptan (Imitrex)

More than 80% of people treated with sumatriptan report significant relief and are usually free of headache after 1 hour.

Miscellaneous Medications

Prochlorperazine (Compazine) can be given intravenously over 10 minutes and may help knock out a headache. Sometimes it causes tightening of the muscles as a side effect, which usually responds to a small intravenous dose of diphenhydramine (Benadryl).

Chlorpromazine (Thorazine) can be given either intravenously or by rectal suppository and tends to make patients sleepy and/or lower their blood pressure.

Rarely do we prescribe opioids, both because they usually do not work well in migraine and are addictive, but they can be tried if all else fails. Injectable opioids such as meperidine (Demerol), should be used no more than twice per month; tablet forms no more than twice weekly. This may be accompanied by promethazine (Phenergan) or hydroxyzine (Vistaril); some centers may administer morphine. Butorphanol (Stadol) can be given by injection or nasal spray. It rapidly relieves pain, may cause drowsiness or dizziness, and does not produce euphoria (a "high").

Antinausea Medications
Refer to page 53 for details.

CLUSTER HEADACHE TREATMENT

If you must go to the emergency room during an attack of cluster headache, the chances are the attack will be breaking by the time you get there. Oxygen inhalation is the most effective and safest treatment. Patients who receive this treatment should be seated, leaning slightly forward; the oxygen mask should fit loosely over the nose and mouth.

Ergotamine tartrate by mouth or under the tongue can be helpful, but injectable dihydroergotamine (D.H.E. 45) tends to work faster. Sumatriptan (Imitrex) injection usually aborts a cluster attack within 5 to 10 minutes.

Pain medication is not specific for cluster headache, but it may decrease the intensity of the pain if nothing else has worked. Cluster patients must not use opiates (narcotics) on a daily basis.

SPECIALIZED INPATIENT THERAPY

When headaches become daily, severe, incapacitating, and when they are associated with disability, decreased quality of life, or rebound syndromes from analgesic and/or ergotamine overuse, aggressive therapy with intravenous medication and cautious withdrawal of the offending medications must begin.

Although treatment can be attempted on an outpatient basis, many patients with severe withdrawal symptoms must be hospitalized, and a well-staffed, properly designed specialty hospital program may yield marked improvement and long-lasting benefits.

Patients who take butalbital-containing medications or opiates everyday are usually best detoxified in a hospital setting to ensure that serious withdrawal symptoms such as epileptic seizures, tremors, insomnia, diarrhea, and incapacitating rebound pain do not occur. If they do, appropriate medical support is available in the hospital.

CONCLUSION

Although we agree that it is preferable to treat patients appropriately on an outpatient basis, our experience has shown us that this is not always possible. Thus, we are convinced that inpatient headache treatment is appropriate and ultimately cost effective under some circumstances.

Children are not immune to headache: the youngest patient to visit our Center was only 3½ years old when she first came to see us. Her mother reported that the child seemed to experience severe headaches since the age of 6 months. She reported that three or four times per year her little girl would become distraught, vomit, and cry inconsolably. The mother noted that the child pressed the same side of her head to her mother's chest each time she had an attack. All medical examinations and tests were completely within normal limits. Between episodes, the child was happy and content. When the child was finally able to describe her pain, it became clear that she was experiencing headache. Migraine was diagnosed at the age of 3½.

Headaches are less common in children than in adults. Studies show that 39% of 6-year-olds get occasional headaches, as do 70% of 15-year-olds and 90% of adults.

CAUSES OF HEADACHE IN CHILDREN

The majority of headaches in children are migraine and/or tension-type headache, rather than headaches due to a serious underlying medical problem. Migraine in children tends to occur more frequently on both sides of the head than on one side, and attacks tend to be shorter than those of adults. Children's attacks can come on much more rapidly and become intense in a short period of time. A child suffering from headache almost always appears pale and ill, and may complain of nausea and then vomit. A child with headache may also exhibit a strong urge to sleep. Although sleep brings migraine relief throughout life, it seems to be especially effective for children.

Children often describe tension-type headache as a mild headache on both sides of the head or as a steady, nonthrobbing, squeezing, pressing, or aching in the forehead or at the top of the head. Occasional headaches such as these should not cause concern; they usually respond to relaxation techniques or small amounts of off-the-shelf medication. We recommend, however, that children under the age of 15 avoid aspirin because aspirin has been associated with Reye's syndrome. We prefer Midrin or acetaminophen. Children may get daily chronic tension-type headache that can be very difficult to treat.

WHEN TO WORRY

Although most headaches in children are not serious, parents should watch for the following danger signs so they can seek medical attention promptly:

1. Headache with fever. This may be due to an infection.
2. Stiff neck and vomiting, with or without fever. This may be caused by meningitis or an inflammation of the covering of the brain and spinal cord. This requires *immediate* medical attention.
3. Fever, confusion, and drowsiness. *Immediate* medical attention is needed to rule out a viral infection of the brain (encephalitis). It is uncommon, but it does occur.
4. Fever, bull's eye rash, history of a tick bite, joint pains, back pain, and weakness on one side of the face or in one arm or leg. These symptoms could signal Lyme disease and should be evaluated immediately because Lyme disease can be cured if treated early.
5. Slowly progressive headache. If a child has headache that steadily worsens over a period of days or weeks, especially if the headache is present early in the morning and associated with drowsiness, visual complaints, nausea, or vomiting, the child should be evaluated immediately. Although it is unlikely for a child to develop a brain

tumor, it must be ruled out if these symptoms are present.

6. Headaches brought on by exertion. Some children complain that they get headaches when they do physical exercise. This is usually benign (not serious) exertional headache or migraine triggered by exercise. Only rarely is this caused by a neurological problem.

7. After head trauma (injury), most children develop brief headaches that disappear within 1 to 2 days. If the headaches are intense, associated with nausea, vomiting, drowsiness, or any other neurological symptoms, the child should be seen by a doctor immediately.

EVALUATION

Although medical conditions may play a role in childhood headache, they do not commonly cause recurrent headaches. Refer to Chapter 2 for information about appropriate examination and testing. Children should be told what to expect from diagnostic tests, which helps to reduce anxiety and encourages them to cooperate.

MIGRAINE "EQUIVALENTS"

Unexplained symptoms that some consider migraine related may be more common in children than in adults. Some children experience unexplained episodes of abdominal pain associated with nausea and vomiting, but no headache. Some doctors believe that these episodes may be caused by the same brain mechanisms that cause migraine and term these pains "abdominal" migraine. Other migraine equivalents may include cyclical vomiting in which children vomit profusely from time to time, but for which no cause can be found.

Finally, we note that our adult migraine patients are much more likely to have had motion sickness and car sickness as children than people who do not suffer from migraine.

PSYCHOLOGICAL FACTORS IN CHILDREN WITH HEADACHE

While psychological factors are not a major cause of headache in most children, they do contribute to it in some cases. If headaches are chronic, or do not respond to the usual treatments, it is appropriate to evaluate the role of stress and social and psychological factors. Children often express their reaction to family conflict through physical complaints. If they are already prone to migraine, they may complain of an increased frequency of headaches.

A small percentage of adolescents experience chronic daily headache. Some studies have shown that adolescents with chronic daily headache who do not respond well to treatment show evidence of depression, which must be treated. A few children have chronic daily headache that responds neither to headache therapy, nor to psychotherapy. Although this pattern is not yet well understood and is difficult to treat, most "outgrow" their chronic headache by the time they complete high school.

Anxiety may play a role in some children's headaches, and our goal is to make their lives as normal as possible. The majority of these children become disabled, they must be tutored at home when their condition becomes severe. Therefore, we ask school officials for flexible programming and to make arrangements for a rest area for time-out as needed, along with any other measures to keep them in school for as many hours as possible.

Families and doctors should cooperate with school officials to help them understand that these children suffer from a biologically based disorder and need understanding and help if they are to overcome it.

TREATMENT

Pharmacologic Treatment

With some exceptions, in general, the medications used to treat headaches in children are similar to those given to adults.

We tend to use an absolute minimum amount of medication—just enough, no more—and rely as much as possible on nonpharmacologic interventions. As with adults, pharmacologic treatments fall into three categories: symptomatic, specific (abortive), and preventive.

Symptomatic therapy. These measures address the pain and nausea and may include off-the-shelf medication, in appropriate dosages and frequency. Children, too, can develop rebound headache and should not take medication on a daily basis for extended periods.

Due to the risk of Reye's syndrome, we recommend that acetaminophen (Tylenol) or ibuprofen (Advil, Nuprin, Medipren) be used instead of aspirin. For more severe headaches, Tylenol with codeine may be used safely on an occasional basis. Antinausea medication should be used as appropriate in small doses. We favor promethazine (Phenergan) by mouth for those who are not vomiting, and by suppository for those who are vomiting. Emetrol is an effective off-the-shelf antinausea medicine.

Abortive agents. When prescription medications are needed for children over the age of 6, our first recommendation is for a combination of isometheptene, dichloralphenazone, and acetaminophen (Midrin), which can be given with or without antinausea medication. Children tolerate this combination well, and the capsule contents can be mixed into a tablespoon of apple sauce for those who cannot swallow capsules. When stronger medications are needed, we sometimes prescribe butalbital, acetaminophen, and caffeine (Fioricet or Esgic), or the same without caffeine (Phrenilin). We often work in cooperation with pediatricians and family doctors to determine what might be best for a given child.

When prescription nonsteroidal anti-inflammatory agents are appropriate, we may prescribe naproxen sodium (Anaprox, available off-the-shelf as Aleve) or meclofenamate (Meclomen). In more severe cases, in children who are 10 or older, we sometimes prescribe small doses of ergotamine (Wigraine tablets).

When migraine is persistent and unresponsive to treatment, some headache specialists give small doses of dihydroergotamine (DHE 45) intravenously, or by injection, to break the cycle. Sumatriptan (Imitrex) is under evaluation for oral and intranasal use in adolescents. We expect sumatriptan and some newer triptans to be approved for adolescents in the future.

Preventive medication. When children have frequent, severe headaches that interfere with their lives, our first line of defense is cyproheptadine (Periactin), an antihistamine available in both liquid and tablet forms, given at bedtime. The majority of children respond well to this regimen, which we decrease or discontinue after 3 to 6 months of successful treatment. We generally reserve use of the tricyclic antidepressants (amitriptyline/Elavil, imipramine/Tofranil) for adolescents, and we prescribe them only in small doses. Beta-blockers such as propranolol (Inderal), nadolol (Corgard), and atenolol (Tenormin) may be effective, as may antiseizure medications such as phenytoin (Dilantin). We may prescribe divalproex sodium (Depakote) for adolescents, but not for younger children to avoid liver toxicity.

Most children with migraine have fewer attacks during the summer, perhaps because their schedules are more flexible without the pressures of school.

Nonpharmacologic Interventions

We try as much as possible to treat headache, especially in children, with nondrug alternatives. Chapter 10, *Treatment without Medication*, reviews many of these techniques.

In children as in adults, we evaluate the role of diet, daily exercise, appropriate rest, and regulation of the sleep-wake cycle; we also look for potential trigger factors. Children who are old enough should maintain their own headache calendars to record their headache frequency and intensities, medication use, and triggers. We try to avoid having the calendars viewed as more "homework," and encourage parents to let their children keep their own calendars. Parents should not focus on one type of trigger or another because undue emphasis, for example, on dietary triggers could cue some children to become "dietary cripples."

Children take very well to biofeedback and seem to enjoy working with the biofeedback computers and care givers. When we notice clear-cut psychological issues or unhealthy family situations, we refer patients and their families for appropriate therapy, but we continue to focus our efforts on the biological aspects of headache disorders. Children's headaches are not "all in their heads" any more than are adults' headaches.

CONCLUSION

Many children have headaches, and most of these headaches are not signs of serious disease. In most cases, a combination of pharmacologic and nonpharmacologic treatments help to relieve headache while enhancing children's quality of life.

HORMONES AND HEADACHE IN WOMEN

Migraine is three times more common in women than in men which is why we have devoted a chapter specifically to women and migraine. Prior to puberty, migraine occurs slightly more frequently in boys than in girls, but after menarche (a girl's first period) its prevalence among women increases dramatically, suggesting that it may be related to female hormones.

Women's susceptibility to migraine increases at the following times: (1) menarche, (2) the start of each menstrual cycle, (3) with use of oral contraceptives, (4) early pregnancy and the postpartum period, (5) the time around menopause (perimenopause), (6) after menopause (postmenopause), and (7) after starting hormone replacement with estrogen and progestins such as progesterone.

The menstrual cycle represents a finely tuned balance between hormones produced by the brain's pituitary gland and the hypothalamus, and those released by the ovaries. The uterus itself produces hormones, prostaglandins, which can cause premenstrual cramps, painful menstruation, and headache. Marked by a rise in estrogen and progesterone levels, ovulation (when eggs are released from the ovaries) occurs at midcycle, usually between the 11th and 14th day of the cycle. Hormone levels begin to drop after midcycle, as shown in Fig. 14–1. When progesterone levels fall, the lining of the uterus sheds and bleeding—menses—occurs. The first day of bleeding is considered day 1 of the cycle.

MENARCHE

Girls become more susceptible to migraine when they have their first menstrual periods; one-third of all women with migraine will experience their first attack within the year after their first period. It appears that the normal cycle of hormones, especially falling estrogen levels, affects brain mechanisms involved in producing migraine.

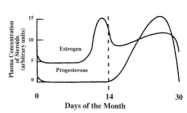

Figure 14–1: The monthly female hormonal cycle (variations of hormone levels during the month).

Menstrual Migraine

According to some experts, menstrual migraine is defined as that occurring between 2 days before a period and 3 days after it starts. Others define menstrual migraine as any headache that occurs at predictable times during the menstrual cycle. Sixty percent of women with migraine have more headaches just before or during their periods. These headaches tend to be the worst attacks of the month and can be the most difficult to treat. Some women report an increase in headache at midcycle when they ovulate (day 13 or 14).

Some of our patients have successfully used estradiol (Estrace)—a synthetic estrogen—placed under the tongue (sublingually) when a migraine occurs during a period. The estradiol may abort the attack, reduce its intensity, or make it more responsive to the usual medications.

Menstrual Migraine Treatment

Treatment of menstrual migraine involves previously discussed pharmacologic and nonpharmacologic interventions. These headaches differ from other migraines only in their timing in the menstrual cycle and that they are triggered by falling estrogen levels just before menstruation.

For women whose headaches occur mostly around menses, we prescribe daily preventive medications, but only for those days leading up to, or during, the projected headache period, rather than throughout the entire month. Refer to Chapter 9 for a description of these medications.

We recommend that patients start preventive medication 5 days before the expected bleeding and continue till it stops. The nonsteroidal anti-inflammatory drugs such as naproxen sodium (Anaprox or Aleve), meclofenamate (Meclomen), flurbiprofen (Ansaid), ketoprofen (Orudis), and ibuprofen (Motrin, Nuprin, Advil, and Medipren) have proven especially useful and should be taken two to three times per day with meals.

We may also prescribe other preventive medications such as cyproheptadine (Periactin), beta-blockers, antidepressants, calcium channel blockers, methylergonovine (Methergine), and methysergide (Sansert). More recently, daily use of bromocriptine (Parlodel) has been prescribed to increase brain levels of a chemical called dopamine.

Hormonal manipulation may help because migraine is induced by falling estrogen levels. Boosting estrogen levels with small doses starting 5 days before menses may prevent or decrease the severity of attacks. Small doses of estrogen given for this purpose generally do not affect the periods. More aggressive hormonal therapy includes agents that block estrogen receptors such as tamoxifen (Nolvadex), and danocrine (Danazol), an androgen (male hormone) that blocks the production of estrogen. Other agents can suppress menses and help headache. It is a good idea to have the doctor who treats your headaches consult with your gynecologist.

Migraine attacks should be treated with standard therapies to abort migraine or lessen the pain (as described in Chapter 9). The focus should be on ergotamine with caffeine (Wigraine), dihydroergotamine (D.H.E. 45), sumatriptan (Imitrex) and the newer triptans such as zolmitriptan (Zomig).

Migraine attacks in women who take oral contraceptives ("the pill") generally occur during estrogen withdrawal, just prior to menses. Sometimes "the pill" needs to be stopped. There is no evidence in the literature that hysterectomy is a reasonable treatment for menstrual migraine.

ORAL CONTRACEPTIVE USE

The effect of oral contraceptives on migraine is controversial. Stephen Silberstein, MD, of Philadelphia, concluded in a published review of the literature that oral contraceptives may worsen or relieve migraine or just change its pattern but that oral contraceptives do not increase the risk of stroke. We believe that if migraines increase in frequency or become more severe when a woman takes oral contraceptives, then it is wise to discontinue their use. If the migraines are stable in a patient who already takes oral contraceptives, we do not suggest that they be discontinued. Women who have migraine with aura, however, should not take oral contraceptives due to a possible increase in the risk of stroke. Smoking, of course, is associated with a much more significant risk of stroke than oral contraceptives. Smokers face a risk of stroke ten times that associated with migraine and oral contraceptives. So, if you smoke and have migraine, particularly migraine with aura, *stop smoking now!*

When oral contraceptives are implicated in migraine, women who discontinue them may not see improvement for 6 to 12 months. Each woman must decide for herself whether a potential improvement in migraine is counterbalanced by the risk of pregnancy or a return of those gynecological symptoms oral contraceptives were prescribed to relieve. If avoiding pregnancy is an issue, other forms of contraception can be considered.

MIGRAINE AND PREGNANCY

As many as 75% of women experience a decrease in the frequency of their migraine attacks during the last 6 months of pregnancy. Migraine without aura is more likely to decrease during pregnancy than migraine with aura. Many women get more headaches during the first

3 months of pregnancy. The frequency of headaches may decrease as pregnancy progresses and estrogen stabilizes at a high level.

We take a conservative position regarding the use of medication during pregnancy; we advise our patients to discontinue all medication prior to getting pregnant. Preventive medications should be discontinued 2 to 4 weeks before attempting to conceive. Since medications that abort migraine should not be used during pregnancy, the only safe time to use them is during the first 10 days of the cycle. Medications that contain ergotamine (Wigraine, and Bellergal) may cause uterine contraction and terminate a pregnancy. Insufficient information is available about the effect of sumatriptan on the uterus or the fetus to justify its use in pregnancy. Potential fathers may want to stop using medications, too.

We prefer that patients use no medication during pregnancy, including any of the standard nonprescription off-the-shelf medication. When, however, medication must be used during pregnancy, we urge our patients to fully discuss possible ramifications with their obstetrician and pediatrician. If medication is necessary, we prefer acetaminophen (Tylenol) to aspirin, particularly during the first 3 months. If more potent medications are required, acetaminophen with codeine, mixed butalbital products (Fioricet), and butorphanol (Stadol) nasal spray (an opiate) are acceptable. Other opiates (narcotics) such as Demerol may be permitted for severe pain. When severe and protracted vomiting occurs, we use antinausea medication such as promethazine (Phenergan).

If attacks occur frequently and preventive medication is necessary, propranolol (Inderal) and verapamil (Calan) may offer a slight margin of safety. As with any other medications, use of preventive agents must be discussed thoroughly.

POSTPARTUM PERIOD

Migraine may return with a vengeance after a baby is born, and it may occur for the first time in some women. Migraine and menstrual periods tend to be delayed in breastfeeding women because estrogen levels remain high as long as nursing continues. We prefer to avoid medication in women who are breastfeeding. Refer to Table 14–1 for medications that should not be used when breastfeeding.

PERIMENOPAUSAL PERIOD

As women approach menopause they may begin to notice subtle changes in the frequency, timing, duration, and amount of flow of their menstrual bleeding. Many women with pre-existing migraine may notice that they get more headaches, perhaps due to fluctuating levels of estrogen and progesterone. A small percentage of women may get their first migraines at this time—whether menopause occurs naturally or due to removal of the ovaries. If you are approaching menopause, be sure to mention your migraine history to your doctor; it may influence the way hormone replacement therapy is implemented.

Many women with migraine do better if they receive hormone replacement on a continuous basis rather than

Table 14–1: Forbidden Headache Medications When Breastfeeding	
Drug Generic Name	Brand Name
Ergotamine tartrate	Cafergot
Lithium	Lithotab
Amphetamine	Dexedrine
Chlorpromazine	Thorazine
Aspirin	Aspirin
Phenobarbital	Phenobarbital

cyclically. If progesterone is appropriate, a low daily dose may be preferable to a high dose 10 days per month.

If you notice that you get more frequent headaches after starting estrogen replacement therapy, you may find that a different estrogen preparation causes fewer headaches.

We recommend nonpharmacologic techniques during menopause, as well as vitamin supplements such as 400 international units of vitamin E and 50 mg of vitamin B6 daily. Recent studies have shown that the use of 400 mg of magnesium may be beneficial. We also suggest 200 to 400 mg of vitamin B2 (riboflavin).

CONCLUSION

Women are more susceptible to migraine than men; their unique needs require special consideration when migraine treatment plans are implemented. For an in-depth discussion of headaches and women, refer to our book, *Headache Relief for Women: How You Can Manage and Prevent Pain*, published by Little, Brown and Company.

CHAPTER 15

TRAVEL, HOLIDAYS, AND HEADACHE

Although holidays are usually associated with good times, family reunions, and happy memories, they bring to some people loneliness, depression, anxiety, and over-commitment—all of which can result in headache in those with the biologic vulnerability. Headache sufferers also have more headaches when they travel.

HOLIDAY HEADACHES

At our Center, we receive up to three times more phone calls during the holiday season between Thanksgiving and New Year's Day than at any other time of year. We attribute this to the combined effects of stress factors and greater exposure to headache triggers such as stress, food, lack of sleep, and over-commitment.

Migraine patients are more affected than others by changes in daily events and body rhythms, and the holidays magnify this susceptibility.

Solutions

The following suggestions should be followed to avoid holiday headaches:

1. Allow an unwinding period after your final day at work and before travel and celebration.
2. Pace yourself realistically; do not overextend yourself; make a schedule that allows you to accomplish a reasonable number of tasks. Do not set unattainable goals.
3. Look for signs of tension such as clenched teeth, tense shoulders, and shallow breathing. When you note them, allow yourself a few moments to relax those muscles and take slow, easy abdominal breaths.
4. Try to sleep the same number of hours every night; try going to bed at a set time and waking up at the same

time. Set specific meal times; do not skip them. Exercise regularly.

5. Remember to take medications as prescribed; do not change dose times. Do not use more than recommended amounts of off-the-shelf or prescription pain medications.
6. Take time to unwind after traveling or holiday activities; ease into your regular routine.

HANGOVER HEADACHE

The hangover headache is a familiar holiday phenomenon that is easier to avoid than treat.

1. Drink very little alcohol and drink slowly, over a period of hours.
2. The lighter color alcohols such as gin, vodka, and white wine tend to have fewer congeners (impurities) and are less likely to cause hangover headache.
3. Use sugar-free mixes to dilute the alcohol and make sure you drink sufficient nonalcoholic liquids.
4. Drink approximately 12 ounces of water for every hour during which you consume alcohol.
5. Before drinking, eat high-protein, more slowly absorbed foods, such as milk or mild cheese.
6. High-fructose food such as apples, honey, grapes, tomatoes, and their juices help you break down (metabolize) the alcohol faster.
7. Stay in a well-ventilated room or go outdoors at intervals for fresh air; avoid inhaling cigarette smoke.
8. Eat bland snacks, avoiding salt and foods that trigger your headaches.
9. Go to bed at a reasonable hour.
10. At bedtime, take 1 to 2 aspirins and drink as much water as possible. Put cold compresses over your forehead, eyes, temples, and/or the nape of your neck.

11. Do not drink alcohol the next morning.

AIR TRAVEL

Anxiety over or the stress of travel can trigger tension-type headache, as can cramped airplane seating conditions. Business- and first-class seating is generally more comfortable than coach class and may be less likely to trigger a headache.

Headache may also occur because recirculated, dry air with decreased oxygen content (or even cigarette smoke) can stress your respiratory system, your brain, and your body's ability to regulate its temperature. Airplane cabins are pressurized to about 7500 feet above sea level; though increased altitude affects many migraine sufferers, it affects cluster headache patients more readily and produces a cluster attack.

Traveling through time zones, especially towards the east, may cause jet lag, which, in turn, may bring on headaches for those who are sensitive to disruptions in their daily schedules of meals, sleep time, and waking time.

The time to start avoiding a travel headache is 24 hours before your flight! Leave plenty of time for all your activities, such as packing, getting to the airport, and checking in. If possible, get your boarding pass in advance so you can go directly to the gate. Try to get an aisle seat so you can get up and walk the aisle every 45 minutes or so. Check bags at curbside where possible; this helps avoid muscle strain due to carrying baggage any farther than necessary. Move around while you wait for your flight—take little walks in the boarding area. While in flight, do gentle neck exercises (as described on page 66) about once an hour.

If you are flying to Europe, you may be able to "reset" your body's clock. Try to get a night flight and go to sleep when the plane takes off; request a blanket if you need one (blinders and ear plugs may help). Your doctor may prescribe zolpidem (Ambien), a relatively new sleeping pill, to help you get to sleep quickly. Melatonin may work for some people, too; take it at your new sleep time.

When your flight lands, try to adjust to the local time immediately: eat and sleep at the locally appropriate times and get a lot of afternoon daylight.

Consider taking headache medication such as Midrin or an NSAID before you leave for the airport and 3 hours later while you are on the plane. Be sure to have headache medications with you in case you develop a severe headache in flight or in a foreign country. Keep medications in their original containers with proper labels and the name of your physician. Some countries may require that you have a letter from your doctor, particularly if you travel with opiates (narcotics) or injectable medications. In addition to medications you normally take for headache, your doctor may want you to have Stadol nasal spray or Decadron tablets on hand as rescue therapy if your usual treatment does not work.

ALTITUDE HEADACHE

Unlike the temporary "altitude" of airplane cabin pressurization, high altitude may be a problem in the mountains. If you spend considerable time at altitudes of 8000 feet or higher you may develop headaches whether you are biologically vulnerable or not.

Reduce your risk of altitude headache by avoiding alcohol, caffeine, and large amounts of pain medication. Be sure to drink sufficient fluids, pace yourself, and take your headache medication as needed. For some patients, acetazolamide (Diamox, 250 mg three times/day) can prevent altitude headaches. Its major side effects include increased urination and tingling in the fingers and around the mouth. We sometimes prescribe dexamethasone (Decadron, 2 to 4 mg up to three times per day for a few days), beginning on the day patients arrive at high altitude; it is relatively safe if used for just a few days.

Acetazolamide, 59, 61, 95
Acetaminophen
  for children, 79, 82
  in combination analgesics, 20
  migraine treatment, 46
  pregnancy, 89
  rebound headaches, 31
  side effects, 4, 39
  tension-type headache treatment,
    37–39, 41
Acupressure, 68
Acupuncture, 2, 68
Advil. *See* Ibuprofen
Air travel, 94, 95
Alcohol, 12, 19, 93–94, 95
Alcoholism, 30
Aleve. *See* Naproxen sodium
Allergies, v, 3, 6, 14
Almotriptan, 51
Alpha₂ adrenoceptor agonists, 58
Alprazolam, 54
Ambien, 94
Amitriptyline, 44–45, 83
Anacin, 39–40, 47
Analgesics
  combination, 39, 40, 47
  rebound headaches, 31–33
  side effects, 4, 39
Anaprox. *See* Naproxen sodium
Androgen, 87
Anemia, 25
Aneurysms, v, 3, 6, 24
Ansaid, 40, 87
Antibiotics, 52
Anticonvulsants, 43, 55, 56
Antidepressants
  menstrual migraine treatment, 87
  migraine prevention, 55
  rebound headaches, 33
  tension-type headache treatment,
    42, 44–45, 46
Antiemetics, 52–53
Antihistamines, 56, 83
Antinausea medication, 38, 44, 51, 82
Anxiety, 21, 23, 29–30
Arthritis, 22
Aspartame, 20
Aspirin
  for children, 82
  in combination analgesics, 20
  migraine treatment, 17, 47
  rebound headaches, 31
  side effects, 4, 39
  tension-type headache treatment,
    37, 49
Asthma, 4, 54
Atenolol, 54, 83
Ativan, 53
Aura, migraine, 6, 8
Autogenic training, 65
Azithromycin, 52

Back pain, 79
Baclofen, 43
Barbiturates, 38
Baskin, Steven, 65
BC-Powders. *See* Analgesics,
  combination
Bellergal. *See* Ergotamine tartrate
Benadryl, 75
Benzodiazepine, 53
Beta-blockers, 33, 54–55, 87
Biofeedback, 34, 66, 84
Blau, Nat, 19

Blocadren, 54
Blood pressure, high, 4, 7, 35, 43
Blood pressure medications, 20
Blood tests, 25
Body scan, 66
Brain
  aneurysms, v, 3, 6, 24
  damage, 13
  tumors, v, 3, 6, 24, 79–80
Breastfeeding, 90
Bromocriptine, 87
Bufferin. *See* Analgesics, combination
Buspar, 53
Buspirone, 53
Butalbital
  for children, 82
  migraine treatment, 47, 52, 56
  pregnancy, 89
  rebound headache, 31, 34
  tension-type headache treatment,
    41–42
  withdrawal, 77
Butorphanol, 43, 52, 76, 89

Cafergot. *See* Ergotamine tartrate
Caffeine
  headache trigger, 20–22, 95
  migraine treatment, 46
  rebound headaches, 31–34
  tension-type headache treatment,
    37–39
Calan, 54, 89
Calcium channel blockers, 33, 35,
  54–55, 58, 60, 87
Calendar, 62–64, 67
Capsaicin, 61–62
Carbamazepine, 55–56
Cardene, 54
Cardizem, 54
Carisoprodol, 43
Catapres, 58
Cerebral palsy, 43
Chiropractic therapy, 2, 68
Chlorpromazine, 53, 75
Chronic paroxysmal hemicrania, 9
Clonazepam, 43
Clonidine, 58
Clorazepate, 53
Cluster headache
  air travel, 94
  emergency treatment, 77
  symptoms, 9, 11–12,
  stress, 28
  treatment, 59–60
Codeine, 31, 38, 41, 79, 82
Coffee, 21, 46. *See also* Caffeine
Cognitive therapy, 66–67
Coital headache, 9
Compazine, 53, 75
Computed tomography (CT) scan,
  25–26
Concentration, impaired, 13, 30
Conception, 91
Contraceptives, oral, 56, 85, 88–89
Cope. *See* Analgesics, combination
Corgard, 54, 83
Coronary disease, 48
Cranial nerves, 18
Cyclobenzaprine hydrochloride, 43
Cylert, 58
Cyproheptadine, 56, 83, 87

Danazol, 87
Danocrine, 87

Darwin, Charles, 1–2
Darwin, Erasmus, 1–2
Decadron, 43, 75, 95
Demerol, 46, 76, 89
Dental problems, v, 6, 12
Depakote, 55, 60, 83
Depression, 23, 29–30
Desipramine, 44
Desyrel, 44
Dexamethasone, 43, 95
Dexasone, 43
Dexedrine, 58
Dextroamphetamine, 58
Diabetes, 54
Diamox, 59, 61, 95
Diarrhea, 7
Diazepam, 43, 53
Dichloralphenazone, 39, 82
Diet, 2, 20, 67
Dihydroergotamine (D.H.E. 45)
  for children, 83
  for cluster headache treatment,
    59–61
  in emergency treatment, 74–76
  migraine treatment, 52
  rebound headache, 34
  use by women, 87
Dilaudid, 42
Dilantin, 55, 83
Diltiazem, 54
Diphenhydramine, 75
Disc disease, 22
Diuretics, 59
Divalproex sodium, 55–56, 83
Dizziness, 7, 26, 41
Doctor-patient relationship, 72–73
Dopamine, 87
Doxepin, 44
Drowsiness, 24
Drugs
  caffeine content, 21
  interactions, 73
  nonprescription, 3–4
Duragesia patch, 42

Ears, ringing in, 4
Elavil, 44–45, 83
Electroencephalogram (EEG), 26
Eletriptan, 51
Emergency headache treatment, 74–77
Emetrol, 53, 82
Encephalitis, 79
Energy, decreased, 13, 30
Epidural patch, 15
Epival, 55
Ergotamine tartrate, 17–18
  for children, 83
  cluster headache treatment, 60, 76
  menstrual headache treatment, 87
  migraine treatment, 51–52
  pregnancy, 39
  rebound headaches, 31, 33
Erythromycin, 52
Esgic. *See* Butalbital
Estrace, 86
Estradiol, 86
Estrogen, 85–87
Excedrin, 3, 20, 39–40, 47
Exercise, 67
Exertional headache, 9
Extremities
  cold, 7
  weak, 24

Eye pain, 11-12,
Eye strain, 14-15

Fainting, 26, 48
Fatigue, 20
Feet, cold, 7
Fentanyl, 42
Fever, 7, 14, 79
Feverfew, 70
Fioricet. *See* Butalbital
Fiorinal. *See* Butalbital
Fish oil, 71
Flexeril, 43
Flunarizine, 54
Fluoxetine, 45
Flurbiprofen, 40, 87

Gabapentin, 556
Garlic, 71
Gastritis, 4
Gastrointestinal bleeding, 40
Ginger, 71
Ginkgo Biloba, 71
Ginseng, 71
Glaucoma, 14, 56
Graham, John, 17
Group therapy, 67

Hands, cold, 7
Hangovers, 93–94
Head injury, 13, 26, 80
Headache
    calendar, 62-64, 67
    causes of, 16-23
    children's, 78-84
    holiday season, 92-93
    psychological factors, 27-30
    rebound, 31-35
    treatment with medication, 36-61
    treatment without medication,
        63-71
    types of, 6-15
    women's, 85-91
Hemiplegic migraine, 48
Herbal therapies, 70-71
Hippocrates, 1
Homeopathy, 70
Hormone therapy, 59, 85, 90-91
Hospital treatment, 74-77
Hydrolyzed fat or protein, 19-20
Hydromophone, 42
Hydroxyzine, 53, 76
Hyperbaric oxygen, 2
Hypothalamus, 23, 85
Hysterectomy, 2, 87

Ibuprofen, 4, 38-39, 82, 87
"Ice cream" headache, 9
Ice pillow, 69
Imipramine, 44, 83
Imitrex. *See* Sumatriptan
Inderal, 54, 83, 89
Indocin, 9, 35, 61
Indomethacin, 9, 35, 61
Infection, 14, 24
Innigran. *See* Sumatriptan
Irritability, 13
Isometheptene, 38, 39, 82
Isoptin, 54

Jaw tension, 22
Jet lag, 94-95
Joint pain, 79

Kadian, 42
Ketoprofen, 39, 40, 47, 87

Kidney damage, 4
Klonopin, 43
Kudrow, Lee, 23

Lamictal, 55
Lamotrigine, 55
Lance, Jim, 19
Laser therapies, 2
Lidocaine, 53, 60,
Light, sensitivity to, 7, 10
Lioresal, 43
Lithium carbonate, 23, 58, 60
Liver, 4, 25
Lopressor, 54
Lorazepam, 53
Lumbar puncture. *See* Spinal tap
Lyme disease, 25, 79

Magnesium, 17, 70, 91
Magnetic resonance imaging (MRI),
    25-26
Marks, David, 61
Massage therapy, 69
Maxalt, 51
Meclofenamate, 40, 83, 87
Meclomen, 40, 83, 87
Medical history, 26
Medipren. *See* Ibuprofen
Melatonin, 95
Memory loss, 13
Menarche, 85-86
Meninges, 18
Meningitis, 3, 7, 24, 79
Menopause, 85, 90-91
Menstrual cycle, 19, 85
Menstrual migraine, 51, 59, 86
Meperidine, 42, 76
Metabolic problems, 25
Metaxalone, 43
Methergine, 57, 60, 87
Methodarbamol, 43
Methylergonovine, 57, 60, 87
Methylphenidate, 59
Methysergide, 59, 60, 87
Metoclopramide, 44, 53
Metoprolol, 54
Midol. *See* Analgesics, combination
Midrin, 33, 46, 79, 82, 95
Migraine, 6–10
    "abdominal," 80
    air travel, 94
    aura, 6, 8
    basilar artery, 48
    causes of, 16-19
    children, 78-80
    cyclical, 58
    diagnosis of, 6-9
    emergency treatment, 74-77
    glaucoma, 14
    hemiplegic, 48
    natural therapies, 70-71
    personality, 27-28
    prevention of, 53-59
    psychiatric disorders, 29-30
    rebound headaches, 31–35
    stress, 28
    symptoms, 24
    tension-type headaches, 22-23
    transformed, 11
    treatment of, 46-59
    triggers, 19-22
    women, 85-91
Migranal, 52, 59
Mineral therapies, 70-71

Monoamine oxidase inhibitors
    (MAOIs), 41-42, 44, 46, 56
Monosodium glutamate (MSG), 19
Morphine, 76
Moskowitz, Michael, 18
Motrin. *See* Ibuprofen
Multiple sclerosis, 43
Muscle relaxants, 43
Muscle tension, 22

Nadolol, 54, 83
Naproxen sodium, 38, 40, 47, 82, 87
Naratriptan, 51
Narcotics, 34, 38, 43, 52, 76, 89, 95
Nardil, 42, 46
Naturopathy, 70
Nausea, 7, 10, 15, 24
Neck, stiff, 24, 26
Neuralgia, trigeminal, 15
Neurological examination, 25
Neurontin, 55
Nicardipine, 54
Nifedipine, 35
Nisoldipine, 54
Nitroglycerin, 20, 35
Nolvadex, 87
Nonprescription drugs, 3-4, 21
Nonsteroidal anti-inflammatory drugs
    (NSAIDs)
    air travel headache treatment, 95
    cluster headache treatment, 59
    menstrual migraine treatment, 87
    migraine treatment, 47, 59
    rebound headache, 31-35
    tension-type headache treatment,
        9, 37, 39–40
Norepinephrine, 59
Norpramin, 44
Nortriptyline, 44
Nose, stuffy, 11
Numbness, 24
Nuprin. *See* Ibuprofen

Occupational therapy, 68
Ondansetron, 53
Opiates, 34, 38, 43, 53, 76, 77, 89, 95
Oral contraceptives, 56, 85, 88
Orgasm, 9
Orudis KT. *See* Ketoprofen
Ovulation, 85
Oxycodone, 42
Oxycontin, 42
Oxygen inhalation, 59, 76

Pain
    abdominal, 80
    chronic, 10-11
    psychogenic, 27
    stabbing, 9
Pamelor, 44
Panic attacks, 29
Parlodel, 87
Parnate, 42
Paxil, 45
Pemoline, 58
Peptic ulcer, 4
Percogesic. *See* Analgesics,
    combination
Periactin, 56, 83, 87
Personality change, 13, 24
Phenelzine, 41, 46
Phenergan, 44, 53, 76, 82, 89
Phenobarbital, 56
Phenytoin, 55, 83

97

Phobias, 29
Photopsia, 8
Phrenilin. *See* Butalbital
Physical activity, 7, 9
Physical therapy, 68–69
Platelets, 17
Post-traumatic headaches, 13
Postpartum headaches, 90
Posture, 22
Prednisone, 60
Pregnancy, 26, 88–90
Procardia, 35
Prochlorperazine, 53, 75
Prodrome, 19
Progesterone, 85, 90
Promethazine, 44, 53,76, 82, 89
Propranolol, 54, 83, 89
Prostaglandins, 59, 85
Protriptyline, 44
Prozac, 42, 45
Psychiatric disorders, 29–30
Psychological factors, v, 3, 27-30
Psychotherapy, 67

Rash, bull's eye, 79
Raskin, Neil, 17
Rebound headache, 4, 11, 31-36, 77
Reglan, 44, 53
Relaxation techniques, 34, 63, 65
Reye's syndrome, 79, 82
Ritalin, 58
Rizatriptan, 51
Robaxin, 43

Sansert, 57, 60, 87
Schoenen, Jean, 71
Scotoma, 8
Sedatives, 31
Selective serotonin reuptake
    inhibitors (SSRIs), 45, 46
Serotonin, 17, 19, 30
Serotonin$_2$ antagonists, 56
Sertraline, 45
Sex headache, 9
Sibelium, 54
Silberstein, Stephen, 88
Sinequan, 44
Sinus problems, v, 3, 6, 12, 14

Skelaxin, 43
Sleep problems, 13, 21, 29
Smoking, 88
Soma, 43
Sound, sensitivity to, 7, 10
Speech, impaired, 24
Spinal tap, 15, 26
Stadol, 42, 52, 76, 89, 95
Steroids, 34, 43, 60
Stomach pain, 4, 41
Stress, 22, 28
Stretching, 69
Strokes, 8
Substance abuse, 30
Sular, 54
Sumatriptan
    for chidren, 83
    cluster headache treatment, 59
    emergency treatment, 75
    menstrual headache treatment, 87
    migraine treatment, 46, 47, 49-50,
        50-51
    use during pregnancy, 89
Sweating, 7

Tamoxifen, 87
Tegretol, 55
Temporomandibular joint syndrome
    (TMJ), v, 12, 15, 22
Tenormin, 54, 83
Tension-type headaches
    causes of, 22,
    children's, 78–80
    migraine, 22-23
    prevention of, 44–46
    symptoms, 10–11
    treatment of, 37-46
Tetracycline, 20
Thorazine, 53, 75
Thyroid, 25
Tick bites, 79
Tigan, 53
Timolol, 54
Tinnitus, 4
Tizanidine, 43
Tofranil, 44, 83
Toprol-XL, 54

Tranquilizers, 31, 39
Transcutaneous electrical nerve
    stimulation (TENS), 70
Tranxene, 53
Tranylcypromine, 42
Trazodone, 44
Trigeminal neuralgia, 15
Trigeminovascular system, 18
Trigger point injections, 69
Trimethobenzamide, 53
Triptans, 47-51
Tumor, brain, 79–80
Tunnel vision, 8
Turin, Allan, 65
Tylenol. *See* Acetominophen
Tyramine, 19, 46

Ultrasound, 68
Urination, frequent, 7

Valerian root, 71
Valium, 43, 53
Vanquish. *See* Analgesics, combination
Verapamil, 54, 60, 89
Vistaril, 53, 76
Visual disturbances. *See* Aura,
    migraine
Visual imagery, 65
Vitamin A, 20
Vitamin therapy, 71, 91
Vivactil, 44
VML 251, 51
Vomiting, 1, 7, 24, 26, 79, 80

Weeks, Randall, 65
Welch, K.M.A, 17
Whiplash, 13
Wigraine. *See* Ergotamine tartrate
Willis, Thomas, 1, 17
Wolff, Harold, 17, 27

Zanaflex, 43
Zithromax, 52
Zofran, 53
Zolmitriptan, 51, 87
Zoloft, 45
Zolpidem, 94
Zomig, 50, 87
Zostrix HP, 61